THE ART OF RADIANCE

The Secrets to Asian Style Skincare

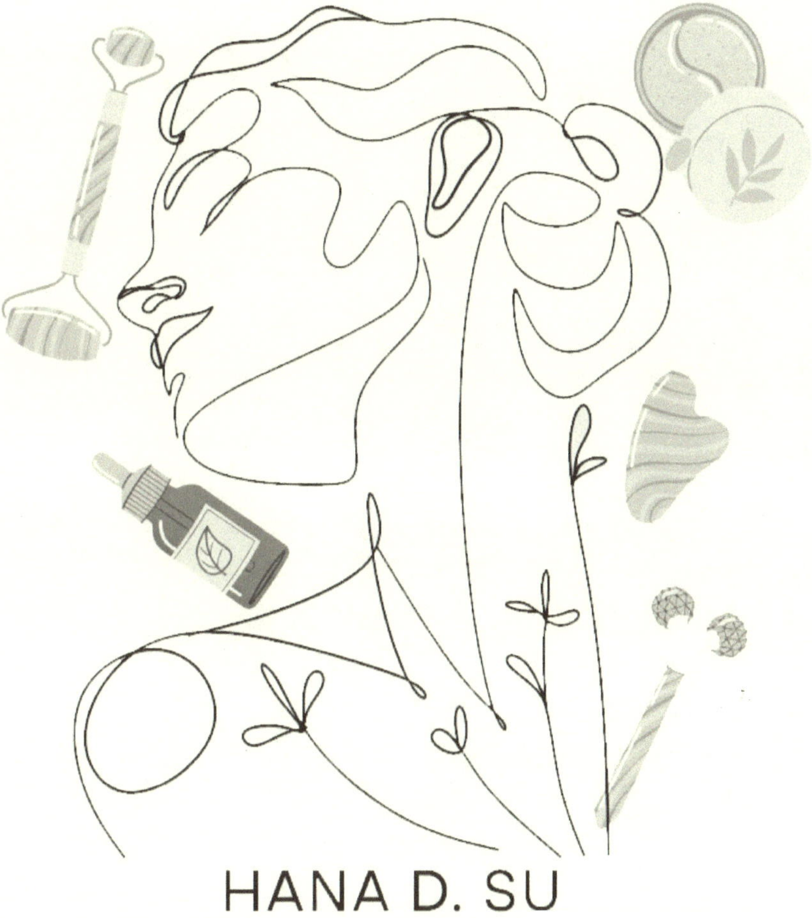

HANA D. SU

TABLE OF CONTENTS

Introduction **9**

The Science Behind the Beauty 10

What You'll Learn 10

How to Read This Book if You Have Limited Time 11

Chapter 1: The Philosophy of Asian Skincare & the Rise of Multi-Step Rituals **15**

The Foundation of Asian Beauty Wisdom 15

The Science of Gentle Care 16

The Multi-Step Revolution 17

Ritualization and Mindfulness 18

The Holistic Approach to Beauty 18

The Future of Asian Beauty Philosophy 19

Chapter 2: Beginner's Routine: Simplifying the Essentials **21**

Starting Your Skincare Journey 21

The Essential 3-Step Foundation 22

Expanding beyond the 3-Step Routine 24

Adapting for Different Skin Types 25

Building Healthy Habits 27

Common Beginner Mistakes to Avoid 28

The Importance of Patience and Observation 28

Chapter 3: Understanding Your Skin **30**

The Foundation of Personalized Skincare 30

The Science of Skin Types 31

Identifying Your True Skin Type 31

Blot Paper Test 34

The Role of Hormones in Skin Behavior 36

Creating Your Skin Profile 36

The Importance of Professional Guidance 38

Chapter 4: Your Skin's Architecture Anatomy, Functions, and the Invisible Ecosystem 40

The Foundation of Beauty: Why Skin Science Matters 40

The Architectural Marvel: Skin's Three-Layer System 41

The Epidermis: Your Body's First Line of Defense 42

The Dermis: The Structural Foundation 46

The Hypodermis: Insulation and Energy Storage 49

The Skin Barrier: A Sophisticated Defense System 51

Chapter 5: Cleansing with Care 55

The Foundation of Healthy Skin 55

The Science of Double Cleansing 56

Understanding Oil Cleansers 57

Water-Based Cleansers: The Second Step 59

Specialized Cleansing Techniques 60

Common Cleansing Mistakes to Avoid 62

The Role of Cleansing in Overall Skin Health 63

Building Your Cleansing Routine 63

Chapter 6: Essences, Toners & Serums 65

The Heart of Asian Skincare Innovation 65

Understanding Toners: Beyond Astringency 66

The Essence Revolution: Fermentation and Innovation....................67

Serums: Targeted Treatment Powerhouses 68

Product Recommendations by Skin Type and Concern....................70

The Future of Essence and Serum Innovation................................71

Chapter 7: Hydration & Barrier Repair: Hyaluronic Acid, Ceramides & Ferments...73

The Science of Skin Hydration 73

Understanding the Skin Barrier...74

Hyaluronic Acid: The Ultimate Hydrator....................................75

Ceramides: The Barrier Builders...77

Climate Adaptation: Hydration Strategies for Different Environments.79

Hydration Techniques 81

Product Recommendations for Different Skin Types.......................82

The Future of Hydration Science...84

Chapter 8: Layering: The Multi-Step Routine from Cleansing to Sunscreen.. 85

The Science of Skincare Layering 85

The Complete Multi-Step Breakdown 86

Additional Optional Steps.. 92

Routine Customization Guide.. 99

Timing and Application Techniques 101

Seasonal Adjustments 101

Building Your Personalized Routine 103

Chapter 9: Power Ingredients: Traditional Wisdom and Modern Innovations 107

Traditional Wisdom Meets Modern Science 107

Ginseng: The Root of Vitality 108

Green Tea: The Antioxidant Powerhouse 110

Rice Water: The Brightening Beauty Secret 111

Aloe Vera: The Plant of Immortality 113

Tea Tree Oil: The Terpinen-4-ol Specialist 114

Calendula: The Gentle Healer 115

Snail Mucin: The Regenerative Marvel 117

Centella Asiatica: The Healing Herb 118

PDRN: The Regenerative Innovation 119

Incorporating Power Ingredients into Modern Routines 120

The Future of Power Ingredients in Beauty 121

Chapter 10: Diet, Lifestyle & Inner Wellness 123

The Holistic Foundation of Asian Beauty 123

The Science of Nutrition and Skin Health 124

The Gut-Skin Axis: Understanding the Connection 125

Stress Management and Skin Health 126

Sleep and Skin Regeneration 128

Exercise and Circulation 129

Hydration and Internal Moisture 130

Creating Your Holistic Beauty Lifestyle 131

Bonus Chapter I: Barrier Health & Probiotic Skincare 133

The Microbiome Revolution in Asian Skincare 133

Understanding the Skin Microbiome 134

Probiotics in Skincare: Living Beneficial Bacteria.......................... 135

Prebiotics: Feeding the Good Bacteria 137

Postbiotics: The Next Frontier... 138

Barrier Function and Microbiome Health 139

Formulation Challenges and Solutions 141

Clinical Evidence and Research... 142

Product Recommendations and Usage Guidelines....................... 143

Integration with Existing Routines.. 144

The Future of Microbiome Skincare 145

Bonus Chapter II: Fermented Extracts & Galactomyces: *The Essence Revolution* 147

The Ancient Art of Fermentation Meets Modern Skincare 147

The Science of Fermentation in Skincare................................... 148

Galactomyces: The Star of Fermented Skincare........................... 149

Other Fermented Yeast Extracts 152

Benefits of Fermented Ingredients.. 153

Formulation Considerations 155

Quality Assessment and Selection.. 156

The Future of Fermented Skincare 157

References...159

INTRODUCTION

The last few years marked a pivotal moment in the global beauty landscape, where Asian style skincare — once considered a niche interest—has evolved into a dominant force reshaping how we approach skin health and beauty worldwide.

Asian beauty and skincare, represents far more than a collection of products or a trending hashtag. It embodies a fundamental philosophy that views skincare as an act of self-care, a daily ritual that honors both the skin's biological needs and the individual's overall well-being. This approach has resonated globally because it addresses a universal desire: the pursuit of healthy, radiant skin that reflects inner vitality and confidence.

As we look into the future of the beauty industry, it is experiencing unprecedented innovation, driven by advances in biotechnology, fermentation science, and personalized skincare. Korean brands continue to lead this charge, introducing groundbreaking ingredients like PDRN (salmon sperm), advanced spicule technology, and sophisticated fermented extracts that were once the exclusive domain of professional treatments.

The Science Behind the Beauty

What sets Asian skincare apart is its unwavering commitment to research and innovation. Beauty companies invest heavily in understanding skin biology, developing new extraction methods, and creating formulations that work synergistically with the skin's natural processes. This scientific rigor has produced ingredients and technologies that are now being adopted globally, from the revolutionary use of fermented extracts to the development of "mirror skin" techniques that surpass even the famous "glass skin" trend.

The Asian approach to skincare is fundamentally preventative rather than corrective. While Western beauty traditions have often focused on addressing problems after they arise, Asian skincare emphasizes maintaining skin health to prevent issues from developing in the first place. The philosophy focuses on both inner wellness and skin health, it looks at the skin as part of the entire human body ecosystem and the goal is to reach a healthy harmonious balance so that the natural rhythm of the body is at work. This philosophy aligns perfectly with current scientific understanding of skin aging, which recognizes that prevention is far more effective than treatment [1].

What You'll Learn

This comprehensive guide is designed to serve as your complete resource for understanding and implementing Asian skincare principles. Whether you're a complete beginner curious about the famous multi-step routine or an experienced enthusiast looking to incorporate the latest innovations, you'll find science-backed explanations, practical guidance, and specific product and ingredient recommendations tailored to your needs.

Each chapter builds upon the previous one, creating a complete education in Asian skincare philosophy and practice. We begin with the foundational concepts and gradually introduce more advanced techniques and ingredients. Throughout, we maintain a focus on the science behind each recommendation, ensuring that you understand not just what to do, but why it works.

The beauty of Asian skincare lies not in its complexity, but in its thoughtfulness. By the end of this guide, you'll have the knowledge and confidence to create a personalized routine that honors your skin's unique needs while embracing the time-tested principles.

How to Read This Book if You Have Limited Time

Think of this book not as a rigid textbook, but as a flexible roadmap to better skin. We understand that life is busy, and diving into a comprehensive guide can feel daunting. That's why we've designed this to be a resource you can use immediately.

Start by focusing on the core principles and actionable steps in the first few chapters. Implement these foundational practices first—getting these right will yield the most significant results. Don't feel pressured to absorb everything at once. Think of it as a roadmap: you can begin with the essentials, implement small but impactful changes in your routine, and gradually build confidence in your approach.

Later, when you're ready to deepen your knowledge and explore more advanced topics, you can return to the book and dive into the chapters you may have skipped. This way, your learning evolves alongside your skincare journey, ensuring steady progress without pressure.

Read Chapter 1 for a foundation of Asian skincare and practices
If you are at a beginner to intermediate level:

- Start with **Chapter 2**, which introduces a simple 3-step foundation to kick off your skincare journey.
- Focus on **consistency over complexity**—a routine you stick to daily will always deliver better results than an elaborate one you can't maintain.
- Start with a simple **skincare journal** to monitor your progress. This can be as straightforward as jotting down the products you use and taking regular photos of your skin over a period of time.
- Treat skincare as a form of **self-care**. Be patient with yourself—visible improvements often take 4–6 weeks of steady effort. Don't forget to celebrate small milestones along the way.
- Highly recommend you make time for **Chapter 10**, which covers diet, lifestyle, and inner wellness. Remember, healthy skin is influenced just as much by what you put into your body as by what you apply on the surface.

If you are at an intermediate to advanced level:

- In addition to Chapters 1–2, dive into **Chapters 3–4** for a well-rounded understanding of the skin's anatomy and how it functions.
- **Consistency is everything.** A steady routine is the foundation of real progress, and using a more detailed **skincare journal** will help you track habits, spot patterns, and notice how different factors impact your skin.

- Prioritize the essentials: **double cleansing** and **daily sun protection**. From there, build your arsenal with proven actives like **Niacinamide, Retinol, and Vitamin C**—ingredients supported by research and effective for a wide range of skin types.

- Explore other chapters based on your personal concerns. For example, if you struggle with **acne** or **pigmentation**, you'll find targeted guidance tailored to these issues.

- Check out **Chapter 8** for a deep dive into building a complete multi-step routine.

- Don't skip **Chapter 10**, which focuses on diet, lifestyle, and inner wellness. Often, addressing lifestyle factors brings more meaningful improvements to your skin than products alone.

- Finally, remember that skincare is a **personal journey of self-care**. Everyone's skin and overall health are different, so adapt what you learn and make it work for *your* unique needs.

If you are at an advanced level and want to know the science:

- Ideally, read the book in its entirety. If time is limited, you can skim through **Chapters 1–3**, but make sure to read **Chapter 4** carefully for a comprehensive understanding of skin anatomy.

- Keep a **detailed skincare journal**, noting all variables that might affect your skin—such as seasonal shifts, environmental changes, and hormonal fluctuations. This level of tracking will help you spot subtle patterns.

- By this stage, you should already have a **well-established, personalized routine**. Focus on refining it by testing new ingredients thoughtfully, rather than chasing every new trend. Your routine should also remain flexible and adaptive as your skin changes.

- Skim **Chapters 5–8** to fill any knowledge gaps. Pay special attention to some key concepts like:

    - Multi-layer skin hydration

    - The skin microbiome and the role of fermented ingredients

    - How the skin barrier functions and how to protect it

- Read **Chapter 9** for insights into these power house ingredients commonly used in Asian skincare formulations.

- Don't miss **Chapter 10**, which covers diet and inner wellness. This topic could fill an entire book on its own, and expanding your knowledge here will greatly enhance your overall results.

- Explore **Bonus Chapter I & II** which are scientific deep dives into two important concepts, **I** for a deeper explanation of skin barrier health and the science behind probiotic skincare, **II** for fermented extracts in skincare formulations and why they can be so transformative.

CHAPTER 1:
THE PHILOSOPHY OF ASIAN SKINCARE & THE RISE OF MULTI-STEP RITUALS

The Foundation of Asian Beauty Wisdom

Asian skincare philosophy represents thousands of years of accumulated wisdom about skin health, beauty, and wellness. Rather than focus on quick fixes and dramatic transformations, Asian beauty traditions emphasize patience, consistency, and the understanding that true beauty emerges from sustained care and attention to detail. This philosophical foundation has shaped modern Asian skincare into a sophisticated system that prioritizes skin health over temporary cosmetic enhancement.

The core principle underlying Asian skincare is the concept of prevention over correction. This approach recognizes that maintaining healthy skin is far more effective and sustainable than attempting to reverse damage after it has occurred. This preventative mindset influences every aspect of Asian skincare, from the gentle formulations that avoid stripping the skin's natural protective barrier to the emphasis on daily sun protection that prevents photoaging before it begins.

Central to this philosophy is the understanding that skin health is interconnected with overall wellness. Traditional Asian medicine has long recognized the skin as a reflection of internal health, and this holistic perspective continues to influence modern Asian skincare. The emphasis on hydration, for example, stems from the understanding that well-hydrated skin is more resilient, better able to repair itself, and naturally more radiant. This is why Asian skincare routines often include multiple hydrating steps, each designed to deliver moisture to different layers of the skin.

The Science of Gentle Care

The Asian approach to skincare is fundamentally gentle, but this gentleness is not synonymous with ineffectiveness. Instead, it reflects a sophisticated understanding of skin biology and the recognition that the skin responds better to consistent, mild stimulation than to aggressive treatments that can disrupt its natural functions. This principle is supported by extensive research showing that maintaining the skin's barrier function is crucial for overall skin health [2].

The skin barrier, composed primarily of lipids and proteins in the stratum corneum, serves as the body's first line of defense against environmental stressors while preventing water loss. Asian skincare formulations are specifically designed to support and strengthen this barrier rather than compromise it. This is achieved through the use of ingredients like ceramides, which help restore barrier lipids, and hyaluronic acid, which provides both immediate and long-term hydration benefits.

Research has demonstrated that gentle skincare approaches are particularly beneficial for sensitive and reactive skin types. A study published in the Journal of Clinical and Aesthetic Dermatology found that patients who used gentle, barrier-supporting skincare products showed significant improvements in skin hydration, reduced irritation, and enhanced overall skin appearance compared to those using more aggressive formulations [3].

The Multi-Step Revolution

The famous multi-step skincare routine stems from solid scientific principles rather than marketing hype. Each step in a comprehensive routine serves a specific purpose, and the layering technique allows for the delivery of multiple active ingredients in a way that maximizes their effectiveness while minimizing potential irritation.

The traditional routine can include anywhere from seven to twelve steps, though modern interpretations often streamline this to a more manageable five to eight steps. The key is understanding that each step builds upon the previous one, creating a synergistic effect that enhances the overall efficacy of the routine. This layering approach is based on the principle of applying products from thinnest to thickest consistency, allowing each layer to penetrate effectively before the next is applied.

The multi-step approach also allows for customization based on individual skin needs and concerns. Rather than relying on a single product to address multiple issues, the method uses targeted treatments that can be adjusted based on seasonal changes, skin condition, or specific concerns. This flexibility is one of the reasons why Asian skincare has proven so adaptable across different cultures and skin types.

Ritualization and Mindfulness

Beyond the practical benefits, the multi-step routine serves an important psychological function by creating a ritualized approach to self-care. The time and attention required for a comprehensive skincare routine can serve as a form of mindfulness practice, providing a daily opportunity to slow down and focus on personal well-being. This aspect of Asian skincare philosophy recognizes that the act of caring for one's skin can be as important as the products themselves.

Research in psychology has shown that ritualized behaviors can reduce anxiety, increase feelings of control, and improve overall well-being. The Asian skincare routine, with its emphasis on careful application and attention to detail, can serve as a form of meditation that helps practitioners start and end their day with intention and self-care. This psychological benefit may contribute to the overall effectiveness of skincare by reducing stress, which is known to negatively impact skin health [4].

The ritualistic aspect of skincare also emphasizes the importance of consistency. Rather than viewing skincare as a chore or a quick fix, the Asian approach frames it as an investment in long-term health and beauty. This perspective encourages practitioners to maintain their routines even when immediate results are not visible, understanding that the benefits of consistent care compound over time.

The Holistic Approach to Beauty

Asian skincare philosophy extends beyond topical treatments to encompass lifestyle factors that influence skin health. This holistic approach recognizes that diet, sleep, stress management, and environmental factors all play crucial roles in skin appearance and health. This comprehensive perspective sets Asian skincare apart from approaches that focus solely on external treatments.

The emphasis on hydration, for example, extends to internal hydration through adequate water intake and the consumption of hydrating foods. Traditional Asian cuisine includes many ingredients that support skin health, such as fermented foods that promote gut health (which is increasingly recognized as important for skin health), and antioxidant-rich vegetables that help combat oxidative stress [5].

Sleep is another crucial component of beauty. The concept of "beauty sleep" is taken seriously in Asian culture, with recognition that the skin's repair and regeneration processes are most active during sleep. This understanding has influenced the development of overnight treatments and sleeping masks that work in harmony with the skin's natural circadian rhythms..

The Future of Asian Beauty Philosophy

As we look toward the future of skincare, the Asian philosophy of gentle, consistent care appears increasingly relevant. Growing awareness of the importance of skin barrier health, the recognition of skincare as self-care, and the desire for sustainable beauty practices all align with traditional approaches to skincare.

The integration of technology into skincare, from AI-powered skin analysis to personalized formulations, represents the next evolution of this philosophy. These innovations maintain the core principles of individualized care and prevention while leveraging modern tools to enhance effectiveness and accessibility.

The Asian approach to skincare offers a compelling alternative to the quick-fix mentality that has dominated much of the beauty industry. By emphasizing patience, consistency, and holistic care, Asian skincare philosophy provides a framework for achieving not just better-looking skin, but a more mindful and sustainable approach to beauty and self-care. As this philosophy continues to influence global beauty standards, it offers the promise of a more thoughtful and effective approach to skincare that honors both traditional wisdom and modern scientific understanding.

CHAPTER 2:
BEGINNER'S ROUTINE:
Simplifying the Essentials

Starting Your Skincare Journey

Embarking on a skincare journey can feel overwhelming, especially when faced with the prospect of a complicated routine and an array of unfamiliar products. However, the beauty of skincare lies not in its complexity, but in its adaptability and focus on skin health. For beginners, the key is to start simple and build gradually, allowing your skin to adjust while you learn what works best for your unique needs.

The beginner's approach to skincare should focus on establishing the fundamental habits that form the foundation of healthy skin: gentle cleansing, adequate hydration, and consistent sun protection. These three pillars, when executed properly with quality products, can deliver remarkable results and provide the groundwork for a more elaborate routine as your knowledge and comfort level grows.

Research consistently shows that consistency trumps complexity when it comes to skincare effectiveness. A study published in the International Journal of Cosmetic Science found that participants who maintained a simple, consistent routine for twelve weeks showed greater improvements in skin hydration, texture, and overall appearance compared to those who used more products inconsistently. This finding validates the philosophy that regular, gentle care produces superior results to sporadic intensive treatments.

The Essential 3-Step Foundation

The most basic Asian skincare routine consists of three fundamental steps: cleanse, hydrate, and protect. This simplified approach captures the essence of Asian skincare philosophy while remaining manageable for beginners and those with busy lifestyles. Each step serves a crucial function in maintaining skin health and can be expanded upon as your routine evolves.

Step 1: Gentle Cleansing

Cleansing forms the foundation of any effective skincare routine, as it removes impurities, excess oil, and environmental pollutants that can clog pores and interfere with the absorption of subsequent products. Asian cleansing philosophy emphasizes gentleness and thoroughness, avoiding harsh scrubbing or stripping formulations that can damage the skin barrier.

For beginners, a single, high-quality cleanser that suits your skin type is sufficient. Look for formulations with a pH between 4.5-6.5, which aligns with the skin's natural acid mantle and helps maintain barrier function. Ingredients like glycerin, hyaluronic acid, or ceramides in cleansers provide additional hydration benefits, while avoiding sulfates and other harsh detergents helps prevent irritation.

The cleansing process should be thorough but gentle. Spend at least 60 seconds massaging the cleanser into damp skin, paying particular attention to areas where makeup, sunscreen, or oil tend to accumulate. This extended cleansing time ensures complete removal of impurities while providing a gentle massage that stimulates circulation and promotes relaxation.

Step 2: Hydration

Hydration is the cornerstone of Asian skincare, reflecting the understanding that well-hydrated skin is more resilient, appears more youthful, and functions more effectively. For beginners, this step can be accomplished with a single, well-formulated moisturizer that provides both immediate and long-term hydration benefits.

The ideal beginner moisturizer should contain humectants like hyaluronic acid or glycerin to draw moisture to the skin, emollients like squalane or ceramides to smooth and soften, and occlusives like dimethicone or petrolatum to prevent water loss. This combination ensures comprehensive hydration that addresses multiple aspects of skin moisture.

Application technique is crucial for maximizing hydration benefits. Apply moisturizer to slightly damp skin, as this helps trap additional moisture and enhances absorption. Use gentle upward strokes, starting from the center of the face and working outward, and don't forget often-neglected areas like the neck and around the eyes.

Step 3: Sun Protection

Daily sun protection is perhaps the most important step in any skincare routine, as UV exposure is the primary cause of premature aging and skin damage. For beginners, choose a broad-spectrum sunscreen with at least SPF 30 that feels comfortable on your skin. Asian sunscreens often incorporate hydrating ingredients like hyaluronic acid or niacinamide, providing skincare benefits beyond UV protection. The key is finding a formula you enjoy using, as the best sunscreen is the one you'll apply consistently every day.

Expanding beyond the 3-Step Routine

Once you've mastered the three-step foundation and your skin has adjusted to the routine (typically after 4-6 weeks), you can consider adding 1-2 additional steps that provide enhanced benefits: a treatment essence and a targeted serum. This expansion aims at adding 1-2 active ingredients at addressing any particular concerns. The goal is to maintain simplicity while introducing the layering concept that is central to Asian skincare.

Step 2.5: Treatment Essence

A treatment essence is a lightweight, watery product that provides an additional layer of hydration while delivering active ingredients to the skin. Essences are applied after cleansing but before moisturizer, and they help prepare the skin to better absorb subsequent products. For beginners, look for essences containing fermented ingredients like galactomyces or bifida ferment lysate, which provide gentle exfoliation and hydration benefits.

The application of essence introduces the technique of "patting" products into the skin rather than rubbing. Pour a small amount into your palms and gently pat it into the skin, allowing each layer to absorb before applying the next product. This technique maximizes absorption while providing a gentle massage that stimulates circulation.

Step 3.5: Targeted Serum

A serum allows you to address specific skin concerns with concentrated active ingredients. For beginners, niacinamide is an excellent choice as it provides multiple benefits including pore refinement, oil control, and brightening effects while being well-tolerated by most skin types. Start with a low concentration (2-5%) and use it every other day initially to allow your skin to adjust.

Serum application follows the same patting technique used for essences. Apply a few drops to skin, pat gently to distribute, and allow full absorption before proceeding to moisturizer. The key is patience—rushing the application process can reduce effectiveness and increase the risk of pilling or irritation.

Adapting for Different Skin Types

While the basic routine structure remains consistent, product selection and application techniques can be modified to address specific needs.

For Oily and Acne-Prone Skin

Oily skin benefits from lightweight, non-comedogenic formulations that provide hydration without adding excess oil. Look for gel-based cleansers with salicylic acid or tea tree oil, water-based essences and serums, and oil-free moisturizers with niacinamide or zinc oxide. The key is maintaining hydration while controlling excess oil production, as dehydrated oily skin often produces more oil to compensate.

Contrary to popular belief, oily skin still needs moisturizer. Skipping this step can lead to increased oil production and barrier damage. Choose lightweight, gel-based formulations that absorb quickly and don't leave a greasy residue. Ingredients like hyaluronic acid and niacinamide are particularly beneficial for oily skin types.

For Dry and Sensitive Skin

Dry and sensitive skin requires gentle, nourishing formulations that strengthen the skin barrier while providing intense hydration. Look for cream-based cleansers with ceramides or glycerin, essences with fermented ingredients, and rich moisturizers with peptides or botanical extracts. Avoid products with high concentrations of acids or alcohol, which can exacerbate sensitivity.

For sensitive skin, introduce new products one at a time and patch test before full application. Start with the most basic routine and add products slowly, allowing at least two weeks between additions to monitor for any adverse reactions. The goal is to build tolerance gradually while providing the gentle care that sensitive skin requires.

For Combination Skin

Combination skin presents unique challenges as different areas of the face have different needs. The T-zone (forehead, nose, and chin) tends to be oilier, while the cheeks and eye area may be normal to dry. Asian skincare's layering approach is particularly beneficial for combination skin, as it allows for targeted treatment of different areas.

Consider using different products on different areas of your face, or adjust the amount of product applied to each area. For example, use a lighter touch with moisturizer on the T-zone while applying more generously to drier areas. This customized approach ensures that each area of your face receives appropriate care.

For Melanin-Rich Skin

Melanin-rich skin has unique characteristics and concerns that should be considered when developing a skincare routine. While melanin provides natural protection against UV damage, it also makes the skin more prone to hyperpigmentation and post-inflammatory marks. Asian skincare's gentle approach is particularly beneficial for melanin-rich skin, as harsh treatments can trigger inflammation and worsen pigmentation issues.

Focus on gentle, hydrating products that support barrier function and include ingredients like niacinamide, vitamin C, and arbutin that help prevent and fade hyperpigmentation. Avoid products with high concentrations of acids or aggressive exfoliants, which can cause irritation and lead to post-inflammatory hyperpigmentation.

Building Healthy Habits

Success with skincare depends as much on developing healthy habits as it does on product selection. Consistency is crucial—it's better to do a simple routine every day than a complex one sporadically. Set realistic expectations and understand that visible improvements typically take 6-12 weeks of consistent use.

Create a routine that fits your lifestyle and schedule. If mornings are rushed, focus on a quick but effective routine that includes cleansing, moisturizing, and sun protection. Save more elaborate treatments for evenings when you have more time to enjoy the process. The key is making skincare a sustainable part of your daily life rather than a burden [6].

Keep a skincare journal to track your progress and identify what works best for your skin. Note any changes in skin condition, new products introduced, and environmental factors that might affect your skin. This record will help you make informed decisions about your routine and identify patterns that might not be immediately obvious.

Common Beginner Mistakes to Avoid

Understanding common pitfalls can help beginners avoid setbacks and achieve better results. One of the most frequent mistakes is introducing too many products too quickly, which can overwhelm the skin and make it difficult to identify what's working or causing problems. Start slowly and be patient with the process.

Another common error is expecting immediate results. Skincare is about long-term skin health rather than quick fixes. While some benefits like improved hydration may be noticeable within days, significant improvements in texture, tone, and overall appearance typically take several weeks to months of consistent use.

Over-cleansing is another frequent mistake, particularly among those transitioning from Western skincare routines. The Asian approach emphasizes gentle, thorough cleansing rather than aggressive scrubbing. Avoid the temptation to cleanse more frequently or vigorously if you're experiencing breakouts, as this can worsen the problem by damaging the skin barrier.

The Importance of Patience and Observation

Asian skincare teaches us the value of patience and careful observation. Your skin's needs will change based on factors like season, stress, hormones, and age, and your routine should evolve accordingly. Pay attention to how your skin feels and looks, and be willing to adjust your routine as needed.

Learn to distinguish between purging (a temporary increase in breakouts as active ingredients accelerate cell turnover) and genuine irritation. Purging typically occurs in areas where you normally break out and should improve within 4-6 weeks. True irritation, characterized by redness, burning, or breakouts in new areas, indicates that a product should be discontinued.

Remember that skincare is a journey, not a destination. The goal is not perfection but rather healthy, resilient skin that looks and feels its best. Embrace the process of learning about your skin and enjoy the daily ritual of self-care that Asian skincare provides. With patience, consistency, and the right products, you'll develop a routine that not only improves your skin but also provides a moment of mindfulness and self-care in your daily life.

CHAPTER 3: UNDERSTANDING YOUR SKIN

The Foundation of Personalized Skincare

Understanding your skin is the cornerstone of effective skincare. Many people operate under misconceptions about their skin type, leading to inappropriate product choices and ineffective routines. Asian skincare philosophy emphasizes the importance of truly knowing your skin—its type, condition, sensitivities, and unique characteristics—as the foundation for creating a personalized routine that delivers optimal results.

The complexity of skin extends far beyond the traditional categories of oily, dry, combination, and sensitive. Modern dermatological understanding recognizes that skin is a dynamic organ that changes in response to internal factors like hormones, stress, and age, as well as external factors like climate, pollution, and lifestyle choices. This dynamic nature means that understanding your skin is an ongoing process rather than a one-time assessment [7].

The Science of Skin Types

Contemporary skin analysis considers multiple factors simultaneously. Sebum production, controlled by hormones and genetics, affects how oily or dry your skin appears and feels. Water content, influenced by barrier function and environmental factors, determines skin hydration levels. Sensitivity, which can be genetic or acquired, affects how your skin responds to active ingredients and environmental stressors. Understanding these factors individually and in combination provides a more complete picture of your skin's needs.

The Asian approach to skin analysis also considers the skin's barrier function, which plays a crucial role in overall skin health. A compromised barrier can make even normal skin appear sensitive or reactive, while a healthy barrier can help oily skin appear more balanced. This understanding has led to the Asian emphasis on barrier-supporting ingredients and gentle formulations that work with the skin's natural functions rather than against them.

Identifying Your True Skin Type

Accurate skin type identification requires careful observation over time rather than a single assessment. The most reliable method involves observing your skin's behavior in its natural state, without the influence of products that might mask or alter its characteristics. This process, sometimes called the "bare-faced test" involves cleansing your skin with a gentle, pH-balanced cleanser and observing how it behaves over the next few hours without applying any products [8].

Normal Skin Characteristics

Normal skin, also called balanced skin, produces moderate amounts of sebum and maintains good hydration levels naturally. It has a smooth texture, small pores, and rarely experiences sensitivity or breakouts. The skin feels comfortable throughout the day without becoming excessively oily or tight. Normal skin typically has a healthy glow and recovers quickly from minor irritations or environmental stressors.

People with normal skin often underestimate the importance of a consistent skincare routine, assuming their skin will maintain its balance naturally. However, normal skin still benefits from proper cleansing, hydration, and sun protection to maintain its healthy state and prevent future problems. The goal for normal skin is maintenance and prevention rather than correction.

Oily Skin Characteristics

Oily skin produces excess sebum, particularly in the T-zone (forehead, nose, and chin). This skin type typically has larger, more visible pores and may be prone to blackheads, whiteheads, and acne breakouts. The skin often appears shiny, especially by midday, and makeup may not last as long due to excess oil production.

However, it's important to distinguish between truly oily skin and skin that appears oily due to dehydration. Dehydrated skin often overproduces oil to compensate for lack of water, leading to an oily appearance that's actually a symptom of inadequate hydration. This distinction is crucial for choosing appropriate treatments, as dehydrated skin needs hydration rather than oil control [9].

Dry Skin Characteristics

Dry skin produces insufficient sebum and often has a compromised barrier function that allows water to escape easily. This skin type may feel tight, especially after cleansing, and can appear flaky or rough. Pores are typically small and barely visible, but the skin may show signs of premature aging due to lack of natural oils and moisture.

Dry skin can be constitutional (genetic) or acquired due to factors like age, climate, or harsh skincare products. Understanding the cause helps determine the most effective treatment approach. Constitutional dry skin requires ongoing support with rich, nourishing products, while acquired dryness may improve with barrier repair and gentler skincare practices.

Combination Skin Characteristics

Combination skin exhibits characteristics of both oily and dry skin in different areas of the face. Typically, the T-zone is oily while the cheeks and eye area are normal to dry. This skin type requires a nuanced approach that addresses different needs in different areas, making it one of the more challenging types to care for effectively.

The Asian layering approach is particularly beneficial for combination skin, as it allows for customized application of different products to different areas. Understanding the specific needs of each area of your face enables more targeted and effective treatment.

Sensitive Skin Characteristics

Sensitive skin reacts easily to environmental factors, skincare ingredients, or physical stimuli. It may experience redness, burning, stinging, or itching in response to products that others tolerate well. Sensitive skin can occur in combination with any of the other skin types, adding an additional layer of complexity to skincare selection.

Sensitivity can be genetic or acquired, and it's important to identify triggers to avoid them. Common triggers include fragrances, essential oils, high concentrations of acids, alcohol, and certain preservatives. Asian skincare's emphasis on gentle, minimal formulations makes it particularly suitable for sensitive skin types [10].

Blot Paper Test

Determining your skin type requires careful observation over a period of time, preferably when your skin is in its "baseline" state without the influence of new products or environmental stressors.

After cleansing your face and waiting 2-3 hours without applying any products, gently press a clean blotting paper onto different areas of your face: forehead, nose, chin, and cheeks. Examine the paper for oil:

- **Oily Skin**: Significant oil in all areas
- **Dry Skin**: Little to no oil in all areas
- **Combination Skin**: Oil in the T-zone, minimal on the cheeks
- **Normal Skin**: Light oil in the T-zone, minimal elsewhere

Symptom Observation

In addition to oil production, observe other indicators:

- **Pore size**: Larger pores typically indicate oilier skin
- **Texture**: Rough or flaky skin suggests dryness or dehydration

- **Reactivity**: Frequent redness or irritation indicates sensitivity
- **Appearance**: Dull skin may indicate dehydration or dead skin buildup

Factors Influencing Assessment

Several factors can temporarily affect your skin's characteristics:

- **Climate**: Humidity increases the appearance of oil; dry air exacerbates dryness
- **Hormones**: Menstrual fluctuations, stress, and age affect sebum production
- **Products**: Active ingredients can temporarily alter skin conditions
- **Season**: Skin may behave differently in summer or winter

For an accurate assessment, observe your skin over several weeks under different conditions. Keep a skin diary, noting how your skin looks and feels at different times of day and under various circumstances.

Professional Assessment

For a more comprehensive analysis, consider a consultation with a qualified dermatologist or aesthetician. Practitioners can use specialized tools such as:

- **Sebum Analysis**: Accurately measures oil production
- **Hydration Measurement**: Evaluates water levels in the skin
- **pH Analysis**: Determines the skin's acid balance
- **Barrier Assessment**: Measures transepidermal water loss

- **Pigmentation Analysis**: Identifies UV damage and pigmentation issues

These assessments can provide valuable information not apparent through visual observation alone, particularly for identifying underlying issues that could affect the effectiveness of skincare.

The Role of Hormones in Skin Behavior

Hormonal fluctuations significantly impact skin behavior, and understanding these patterns helps predict and manage skin changes. Women may notice that their skin becomes oilier or more prone to breakouts during certain phases of their menstrual cycle, while pregnancy, menopause, and other hormonal changes can dramatically alter skin characteristics [11].

A gentle, adaptable approach is particularly beneficial for managing hormonal skin changes. Rather than using harsh treatments that might work against hormonal fluctuations, it's important to support the skin through these changes with consistent, gentle care that can be adjusted as needed.

Stress hormones like cortisol also significantly impact skin health, affecting everything from oil production to barrier function to healing capacity. Using skincare as self-care and stress relief can help address both the direct effects of stress on skin and the underlying stress itself.

Creating Your Skin Profile

Developing a comprehensive understanding of your skin involves creating a detailed skin profile that goes beyond basic type classification. This profile should include your skin type, specific concerns, sensitivity levels, hormonal patterns, seasonal variations, and response to different ingredients and environmental factors.

Keep a skin diary to track patterns and changes over time. Note how your skin responds to new products, environmental changes, stress, diet modifications, and hormonal fluctuations. This information becomes invaluable for making informed decisions about your skincare routine and identifying what works best for your unique skin.

Your skin profile should be a living document that evolves as you learn more about your skin and as your skin changes over time. Regular reassessment ensures that your skincare routine remains appropriate and effective as your needs change.

To create a comprehensive skin profile, you should include:

Base Characteristics

- Primary skin type (oily, dry, combination, normal)
- Sensitivity level
- Skin tone and related concerns
- Seasonal trends

Current Concerns

- Immediate concerns (acne, dryness, sensitivity)
- Long-term goals (anti-aging, brightening)
- Specific problem areas

Influencing factors

- Hormonal patterns
- Lifestyle factors (stress, diet, sleep)
- Environmental exposure
- Product history

Ingredient Responses

- Ingredients that have worked well
- Ingredients that have caused irritation
- Tolerated concentrations %
- Preferred application methods

This profile serves as a roadmap for product selection and routine development and should be updated regularly as your skin changes and your routine evolves.

The Importance of Professional Guidance

While self-assessment is valuable, professional guidance can provide information not apparent through personal observation. Dermatologists can identify underlying medical conditions affecting the skin, while qualified aestheticians can provide detailed skin analysis and product recommendations.

Consider professional consultation if:

- You experience sudden changes in skin behavior
- You have persistent concerns that don't respond to home care

- You are considering more aggressive treatments
- You have specific skin conditions that require specialized management

The combination of self-awareness and professional guidance provides the strongest foundation for developing an effective and sustainable skincare routine that evolves with your changing needs. Understanding your skin is an ongoing journey rather than a destination. As you develop this understanding, you'll become more confident in making skincare decisions and more skilled at adapting your routine to meet your skin's changing needs.

CHAPTER 4:
YOUR SKIN'S ARCHITECTURE
Anatomy, Functions, and the Invisible Ecosystem

The Foundation of Beauty: Why Skin Science Matters

Understanding the intricate architecture of human skin represents the cornerstone of effective skincare, particularly within the Asian beauty philosophy that emphasizes working with rather than against the skin's natural processes. The skin, as the body's largest organ, functions as far more than a simple protective covering—it serves as a complex, dynamic ecosystem that houses trillions of beneficial microorganisms while maintaining sophisticated barrier functions that determine overall skin health and appearance.

Modern dermatological research has revolutionized our understanding of skin structure and function, revealing that what we see on the surface represents only a fraction of the complex biological processes occurring within the skin's multiple layers. Asian skincare's success stems largely from its recognition of these underlying processes, developing formulations and techniques that support rather than disrupt the skin's natural architecture and microbial balance [12].

The integration of traditional Asian wisdom with contemporary skin science has created an approach that honors the skin's complexity while providing practical solutions for maintaining optimal skin health. This chapter explores the fundamental architecture of human skin, the specialized functions of each layer, and the remarkable microbial ecosystem that calls our skin home, providing the scientific foundation necessary for understanding why Asian skincare methods are so effective across diverse skin types and concerns.

The Architectural Marvel: Skin's Three-Layer System

Human skin represents one of nature's most sophisticated architectural achievements, consisting of three distinct yet interconnected layers that work in harmony to protect, regulate, and maintain the body's internal environment. Each layer possesses unique structural characteristics and specialized functions that contribute to overall skin health and appearance, creating a complex system that requires careful consideration in any effective skincare approach.

The epidermis, dermis, and hypodermis each play crucial roles in maintaining skin integrity, with their interactions determining everything from moisture retention and barrier function to aging patterns and response to skincare treatments. Understanding these layers and their functions provides the foundation for making informed decisions about skincare ingredients, application techniques, and routine customization that aligns with Asian beauty principles.

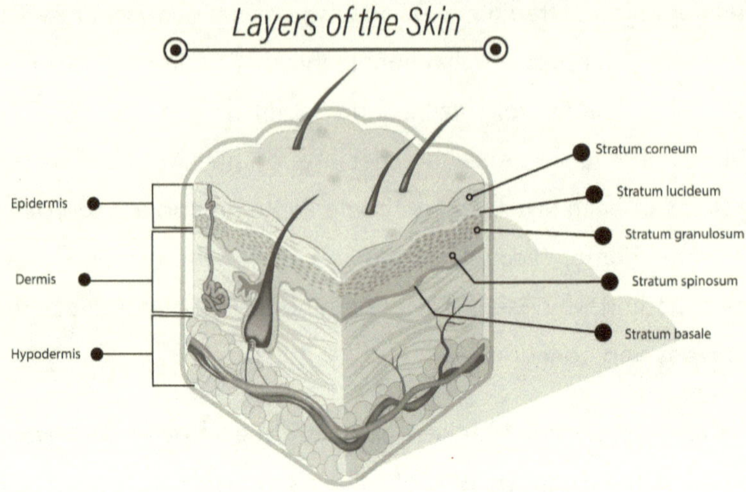

The Epidermis: Your Body's First Line of Defense

The epidermis represents the outermost layer of skin, serving as the primary interface between the internal body environment and the external world. Despite being only 0.05 to 1.5 millimeters thick depending on body location, the epidermis performs multiple critical functions that determine skin health, appearance, and response to environmental stressors.

Structural Organization and Cellular Architecture

The epidermis consists of five distinct sublayers, each representing different stages of cellular development and keratinization. The deepest layer, the stratum basale, contains actively dividing keratinocytes that continuously produce new skin cells. These cells begin their journey upward through the epidermis, undergoing progressive changes in structure and function as they migrate toward the surface [13].

The stratum spinosum, or "spiny layer," contains keratinocytes connected by desmosomes, creating a strong intercellular network that provides structural integrity. As cells continue their upward migration, they enter the stratum granulosum, where they begin producing keratohyalin granules containing proteins essential for barrier function. The stratum lucidum, present only in thick skin areas like palms and soles, provides additional protection in high-stress areas.

The outermost layer, the stratum corneum, consists of flattened, dead keratinocytes called corneocytes embedded in a lipid matrix. This layer, often compared to a "brick and mortar" structure, provides the primary barrier function that prevents water loss and protects against environmental threats. The stratum corneum undergoes constant renewal, with the entire layer replacing itself approximately every 28 days in healthy young adults [14].

Barrier Function and Permeability Control

The epidermis's most critical function involves maintaining the permeability barrier that regulates water loss and prevents the entry of harmful substances. This barrier function primarily resides in the stratum corneum (outer layer of the skin), where specialized lipids including ceramides, cholesterol, and free fatty acids create a hydrophobic barrier that retards transcutaneous water loss while maintaining skin hydration [15].

The barrier function operates through multiple mechanisms, including the physical structure of corneocytes and intercellular lipids, the chemical composition of barrier lipids, and the regulation of desquamation processes that control how dead skin cells are shed from the surface. Disruption of any of these mechanisms can lead to barrier dysfunction, resulting in increased sensitivity, dryness, and susceptibility to irritation.

Asian skincare's emphasis on gentle cleansing and barrier support reflects an understanding of the delicate nature of epidermal barrier function.

Harsh treatments that strip natural lipids or disrupt the pH balance can compromise barrier integrity, leading to a cascade of problems including increased inflammation, enhanced penetration of irritants, and accelerated aging processes.

Immune Function and Langerhans Cells

The epidermis houses specialized immune cells called Langerhans cells that serve as sentinels, detecting and responding to potential threats. These dendritic cells represent approximately 2-4% of epidermal cells and play crucial roles in both innate and adaptive immune responses. Langerhans cells capture antigens that penetrate the skin barrier and present them to T-cells, initiating appropriate immune responses.

The distribution and function of Langerhans cells can be influenced by various factors including UV exposure, age, and skincare practices. Chronic inflammation or barrier disruption can alter Langerhans cell function, potentially contributing to increased sensitivity or altered immune responses. Focus on anti-inflammatory ingredients and gentle treatment approaches helps maintain optimal Langerhans cell function [16].

Melanocyte Function and Pigmentation Control

Melanocytes, located in the basal layer of the epidermis, produce melanin pigment that provides natural protection against UV radiation while determining skin color. These specialized cells extend dendritic processes to surrounding keratinocytes, transferring melanin-containing organelles called melanosomes that provide photoprotection.

The melanin production process, known as melanogenesis, involves complex biochemical pathways regulated by multiple factors including UV exposure, hormones, and inflammatory mediators. Understanding melanogenesis is crucial for addressing hyperpigmentation concerns, particularly in melanin-rich skin where post-inflammatory hyperpigmentation represents a common concern.

Asian skincare's approach to pigmentation management emphasizes prevention through gentle care and consistent sun protection, recognizing that inflammation can trigger unwanted melanin production. It uses gentle brightening ingredients that work with rather than against natural melanogenesis processes because of epidermal melanocyte function.

Implications for Skin Care

Understanding the structure and function of the epidermis has several practical implications for skin care:

1. **Importance of the Barrier Function:** Many skin problems can be traced back to compromised barrier function. Products that support the barrier—those containing ceramides, hyaluronic acid, or ingredients that maintain proper pH—are critical for skin health.

2. **Cell Renewal:** Ingredients that promote healthy cell renewal, such as mild acids or enzymes, can improve skin texture and appearance. However, these should be used judiciously to avoid over-exfoliation.

3. **Pigmentation Protection:** Understanding how melanogenesis works helps explain why prevention (through sun protection and anti-inflammatory ingredients) is more effective than treatment for pigmentation problems.

4. **pH**: Using products that maintain the skin's natural pH helps preserve the barrier function and prevent irritation.

The Dermis: The Structural Foundation

The dermis, located beneath the epidermis, is significantly thicker (typically 1–4 millimeters) and serves as the structural foundation of the skin. This layer is responsible for the skin's strength, elasticity, and youthful appearance. Understanding the dermis is crucial to understanding skin aging and how various anti-aging treatments work to maintain or restore dermal function.

Collagen and Elastin: The Structural Proteins

The dermis consists primarily of collagen and elastin fibers embedded in a ground substance of glycosaminoglycans and proteoglycans. Collagen, representing approximately 70% of dermal dry weight, provides tensile strength and structural integrity. Type I collagen predominates in the dermis, with smaller amounts of types III, V, and VII collagen contributing to specific structural functions.

Elastin fibers, comprising 2-4% of dermal dry weight, provide the elasticity that allows skin to return to its original shape after stretching or deformation. The arrangement and quality of elastin fibers determine skin's ability to maintain firmness and resist sagging. Age-related changes in both collagen and elastin contribute significantly to visible aging signs including wrinkles, loss of firmness, and decreased resilience.

The synthesis and maintenance of dermal collagen and elastin depend on fibroblast activity, which can be influenced by various factors including UV exposure, inflammation, hormonal changes, and nutritional status. Asian skincare generally emphasizes ingredients that support collagen synthesis, such as peptides, vitamin C, and growth factors. There is also a focus on consuming food that facilitates collagen production such as fish, eggs, bone broth, etc. The consumption of sufficient vitamin C and zinc are also critical to collagen synthesis.

Vascular Network and Nutrient Delivery

The dermis contains an extensive vascular network organized into superficial and deep plexuses that supply nutrients to both dermal and epidermal cells. The superficial vascular plexus, located just beneath the dermal-epidermal junction, provides nutrients to the metabolically active basal layer of the epidermis through diffusion.

Blood flow regulation in dermal vessels plays crucial roles in temperature regulation, wound healing, and inflammatory responses. Factors that improve dermal circulation, including massage, certain skincare ingredients, and lifestyle factors, can enhance nutrient delivery and support overall skin health. It's very helpful to incorporate facial massage techniques such as Gua-Sha and circulation-enhancing ingredients like ginseng. The traditional Asian belief is to use a natural stone material such as jade for the Gua-Sha tool and jade is believed to have beneficial energies for the human body, there is no scientific study to back these traditional claims, any material should work just fine.

The dermal vascular network also plays important roles in the delivery of topically applied skincare ingredients. Understanding vascular anatomy helps explain why certain application techniques and ingredient combinations may be more effective.

Appendageal Structures: Hair Follicles and Glands

The dermis houses important appendageal structures including hair follicles, sebaceous glands, and sweat glands that significantly influence skin function and appearance. Hair follicles extend from the epidermis deep into the dermis, with associated sebaceous glands producing sebum that contributes to skin barrier function and antimicrobial protection.

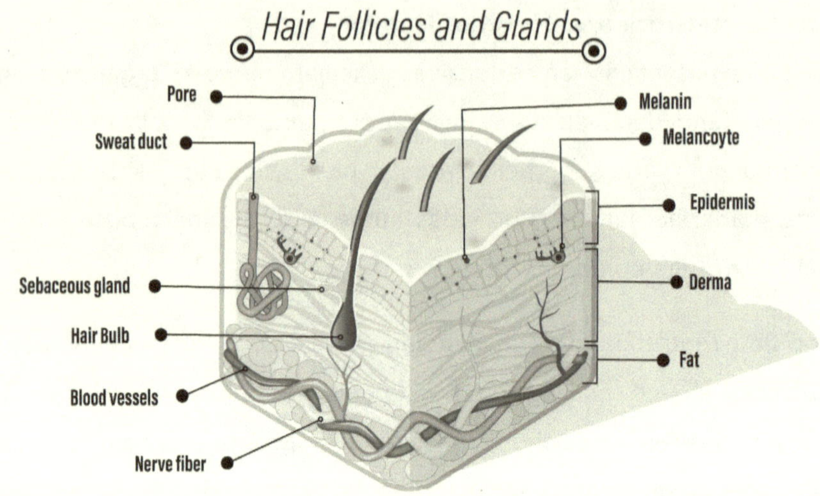

Sebaceous glands produce sebum, a complex mixture of lipids including triglycerides, wax esters, squalene, and cholesterol esters. Sebum production is regulated by hormones, particularly androgens, and varies significantly between individuals and body sites. Understanding sebum composition and regulation is crucial for managing oily skin and acne-prone conditions.

Eccrine sweat glands, distributed throughout the body, produce sweat that aids in temperature regulation and contributes to skin surface pH and antimicrobial protection. Apocrine glands, located primarily in axillary and genital areas, produce a different type of secretion that can influence skin microbiome composition. pH balance and gentle cleansing are good practices for these glandular structures.

Implications for Skin Care

Understanding dermal structure and function informs several skin care strategies:

1. **Collagen Stimulation:** Ingredients that stimulate collagen synthesis (such as retinoids, vitamin C, and peptides) can help maintain skin firmness

2. **Antioxidant Protection:** Antioxidants help protect the ECM from oxidative damage that can accelerate aging

3. **Hydration:** Maintaining dermal hydration through humectants like hyaluronic acid supports overall skin function

4. **Sun Protection:** Preventing UV damage protects both collagen and elastin from degradation

5. **Anti-inflammatory Ingredients:** Reducing chronic inflammation helps preserve fibroblast function and the integrity of the ECM

The Hypodermis: Insulation and Energy Storage

The hypodermis, also known as the subcutaneous layer, represents the deepest layer of skin and serves multiple functions including insulation, energy storage, and mechanical protection. This layer consists primarily of adipose tissue organized into lobules separated by fibrous septa that connect the dermis to underlying muscle and fascia.

Tissue Organization and Function

Subcutaneous adipose tissue is organized into distinct lobules containing mature adipocytes (fat cells) along with preadipocytes, fibroblasts, immune cells, and an extensive vascular network. The thickness of the hypodermis varies significantly between body sites and individuals, influenced by factors including genetics, age, sex, and nutritional status.

The adipocytes in the hypodermis serve multiple functions beyond simple energy storage. They produce hormones and cytokines that influence metabolism, inflammation, and immune function. Leptin, produced by adipocytes, regulates appetite and energy expenditure while also influencing immune responses and wound healing processes.

Age-related changes in subcutaneous fat distribution contribute significantly to facial aging, with volume loss in specific areas leading to sagging, hollowing, and altered facial contours. Understanding these changes helps explain why Asian skincare emphasizes prevention and maintenance of skin structure through consistent, gentle care rather than aggressive interventions [17].

Mechanical Protection and Shock Absorption

The hypodermis provides mechanical protection for underlying structures, cushioning muscles and bones from external trauma. This protective function is particularly important in areas subject to pressure or friction, where adequate subcutaneous padding helps prevent injury and maintains skin integrity.

The mechanical properties of the hypodermis influence skin texture and appearance, with adequate subcutaneous support contributing to smooth, youthful-looking skin. Age-related changes in subcutaneous structure can affect skin texture and may contribute to the development of cellulite and other textural irregularities.

The Skin Barrier: A Sophisticated Defense System

The skin barrier represents one of the most sophisticated biological defense systems, protecting the body from environmental threats while maintaining internal homeostasis. This barrier function involves multiple components working in concert, including physical barriers, chemical barriers, immunological barriers, and microbial barriers that together create a comprehensive protective system [18].

Physical Barrier Components

The physical barrier primarily resides in the stratum corneum, where corneocytes embedded in lipid lamellae create a structure often compared to bricks and mortar. The corneocytes, derived from terminally differentiated keratinocytes, are surrounded by a cornified envelope composed of cross-linked proteins that provide structural integrity.

The intercellular lipid lamellae, consisting primarily of ceramides, cholesterol, and free fatty acids, fill the spaces between corneocytes and provide the primary barrier to water loss and penetration of external substances. The organization of these lipids into lamellar bilayers creates a tortuous pathway that effectively impedes the movement of water and other molecules [19].

The physical barrier's effectiveness depends on proper lipid composition, organization, and renewal. Factors that disrupt lipid synthesis, organization, or removal can compromise barrier function, leading to increased permeability, sensitivity, and susceptibility to irritation.

Chemical Barrier Functions

The skin's chemical barrier involves multiple components including pH regulation, antimicrobial peptide production, and antioxidant systems that protect against chemical and biological threats. The skin surface maintains an acidic pH, typically between 4.5-5.5, that inhibits the growth of pathogenic microorganisms while supporting beneficial bacteria.

The acid mantle, created by the combination of sebum, sweat, and desquamated corneocytes, provides chemical protection against pathogens and helps maintain optimal conditions for barrier function. Disruption of skin pH can compromise both barrier function and antimicrobial protection, highlighting the importance of pH-balanced skincare products [20].

Antimicrobial peptides, including defensins, cathelicidins, and other compounds, are produced by keratinocytes and provide chemical defense against pathogens. These peptides can be upregulated in response to barrier disruption or infection, representing an important adaptive response to threats.

Immunological Barrier Components

The skin's immunological barrier involves both innate and adaptive immune components that detect and respond to potential threats. Langerhans cells in the epidermis serve as antigen-presenting cells, capturing and processing antigens for presentation to T-cells in regional lymph nodes.

Keratinocytes themselves participate in immune responses through the production of cytokines, chemokines, and antimicrobial peptides in response to various stimuli. This innate immune function allows the skin to mount rapid responses to potential threats while also communicating with systemic immune systems.

The skin-associated lymphoid tissue (SALT) represents a specialized component of the immune system that includes resident and circulating immune cells in the skin. Understanding these immune functions helps explain why gentle skincare approaches that avoid triggering unnecessary inflammatory responses are generally more effective for long-term skin health.

Barrier Function and Product Penetration

Understanding barrier function also helps explain how skin care products penetrate the skin and exert their effects. The intact skin barrier is selectively permeable—it allows certain substances to pass through while blocking others. Factors that influence penetration include:

1. **Molecular Size:** Smaller molecules generally penetrate better than larger ones

2. **Lipid Solubility:** Substances that are soluble in lipids can more easily pass through intercellular lipids

3. **pH:** The pH of the product can affect both the stability of the ingredient and the permeability of the barrier

4. **Concentration:** Higher concentrations generally result in greater penetration

5. **Formulation Vehicle:** The delivery system can significantly affect penetration

Barrier Dysfunction and Skin Problems

Many common skin problems can be traced to compromised barrier function:

1. **Dry Skin:** Often results from increased transepidermal water loss due to compromised barrier function

2. **Sensitive Skin:** Can result from a compromised barrier that allows irritants to penetrate more easily

3. **Dermatitis:** Many forms of dermatitis involve barrier dysfunction as a primary or contributing factor

4. **Acne:** Although traditionally viewed as a problem of clogged pores, research suggests that barrier dysfunction may contribute to the development of acne

Maintaining a Healthy Barrier

1. **Gentle Cleansing:** Avoid stripping products that can damage barrier lipids

2. **Proper Hydration:** Use products containing moisturizers, emollients, and occlusives

3. **pH Maintenance:** Use products that respect the skin's natural pH

4. **Sun Protection:** Prevent UV damage that can compromise barrier function

5. **Avoid Over-Exfoliation:** Excessive exfoliation can damage the skin barrier

6. **Barrier Repair Ingredients:** Use products containing ceramides, hyaluronic acid, and other ingredients that support barrier function

CHAPTER 5:
CLEANSING WITH CARE

The Foundation of Healthy Skin

Cleansing represents the cornerstone of any effective skincare routine, yet it remains one of the most misunderstood and improperly executed steps in many people's daily regimens. Asian skincare philosophy approaches cleansing as both an art and a science, emphasizing thoroughness without aggression, effectiveness without damage, and the understanding that proper cleansing sets the stage for everything that follows in your skincare routine.

The Asian approach to cleansing does not prioritize the feeling of "squeaky clean" skin. Instead, Asian cleansing philosophy focuses on removing impurities while maintaining the skin's natural protective barrier and optimal pH balance. This approach recognizes that the skin's acid mantle plays a crucial role in defending against harmful bacteria, environmental pollutants, and moisture loss.

Research has consistently shown that aggressive cleansing can disrupt the skin barrier, leading to increased sensitivity, dryness, inflammation, and even accelerated aging. A study published in the International Journal of

Cosmetic Science demonstrated that participants who used gentle, pH-balanced cleansers showed significant improvements in skin barrier function, hydration levels, and overall skin health compared to those using traditional alkaline soaps. This scientific validation supports the emphasis on gentle, respectful cleansing practices [21].

The Science of Double Cleansing

Double cleansing, perhaps the most famous aspect of Asian skincare, is based on the fundamental chemical principle that "like dissolves like." This two-step process uses an oil-based cleanser followed by a water-based cleanser to ensure complete removal of all types of impurities that accumulate on the skin throughout the day.

The first step, oil cleansing, is designed to dissolve and remove oil-based impurities including makeup, sunscreen, sebum, and environmental pollutants. These substances are not effectively removed by water-based cleansers alone, as oil and water naturally repel each other. Oil cleansers work by dissolving these oil-based impurities, making them easy to rinse away when the oil is emulsified with water.

The second step uses a water-based cleanser to remove any remaining impurities, including sweat, dirt, bacteria, and water-based products. This step also ensures complete removal of the oil cleanser, leaving the skin perfectly clean and prepared for subsequent skincare products. The double cleansing method has been shown to be significantly more effective at removing impurities than single cleansing alone, while being gentler on the skin than aggressive scrubbing or harsh detergents.

Understanding Oil Cleansers

Modern oil cleansers are sophisticated formulations that bear little resemblance to the heavy, greasy oils that some people imagine. These products are carefully formulated with emulsifiers that allow them to transform from oil to milk when mixed with water, making them easy to rinse off completely without leaving any residue.

Types of Oil Cleansers

Pure oils, such as jojoba, sweet almond, or grapeseed oil, can be used for oil cleansing, but they require more effort to remove completely and may not be suitable for all skin types. Commercial oil cleansers are formulated with emulsifiers like PEG-20 glyceryl triisostearate, polysorbate 80, or sorbitan sesquioleate that ensure easy removal while maintaining cleansing effectiveness.

Cleansing balms are solid oil cleansers that melt upon contact with skin temperature. They often contain additional beneficial ingredients like antioxidants, botanical extracts, or vitamins. Balms tend to be richer and more nourishing than liquid oil cleansers, making them particularly suitable for dry or mature skin.

Cleansing oils come in liquid form and are typically lighter in texture than balms. They're often preferred by those with oily or combination skin, as they feel less heavy on the skin while still providing effective cleansing. Many cleansing oils incorporate lightweight oils like squalane or caprylic/capric triglyceride that cleanse effectively without feeling greasy.

Choosing the Right Oil Cleanser

The key to selecting an appropriate oil cleanser lies in understanding your skin type and specific needs. Those with sensitive skin should look for cleansers with minimal ingredients and avoid products containing essential oils or strong fragrances that might cause irritation. Oily skin types can benefit from cleansers containing ingredients like tea tree oil or salicylic acid that provide additional pore-cleansing benefits.

For those wearing heavy makeup or waterproof products, a more robust oil cleanser with stronger dissolving power may be necessary. Conversely, those who wear minimal makeup or spend most of their time indoors may find that a gentler formulation is sufficient for their needs.

Proper Oil Cleansing Technique

The effectiveness of oil cleansing depends as much on technique as it does on product selection. Begin with completely dry hands and a dry face, as water can interfere with the oil's ability to dissolve oil-based impurities. Apply the oil cleanser generously—using too little product reduces effectiveness and can require more rubbing, which can irritate the skin.

Massage the oil cleanser into the skin using gentle, circular motions for 1-2 minutes. Pay particular attention to areas where makeup, sunscreen, or oil tend to accumulate, such as around the nose, in the T-zone, and along the hairline. The massage should be thorough but gentle—there's no need for aggressive rubbing or pressure.

When ready to remove the cleanser, wet your hands with lukewarm water and gently massage the oil again. This step emulsifies the oil, turning it milky white and allowing it to rinse away easily. Continue massaging with wet hands for 30-60 seconds, then rinse thoroughly with lukewarm water. The skin should feel clean but not tight or stripped.

Water-Based Cleansers: The Second Step

The second step of double cleansing uses a water-based cleanser to ensure complete removal of all impurities and any residue from the oil cleanser. This step is crucial for preparing the skin to absorb subsequent skincare products effectively and maintaining optimal skin health.

Types of Water-Based Cleansers

Gel cleansers are typically clear or translucent and have a lightweight, refreshing feel. They're often preferred by those with oily or combination skin, as they provide thorough cleansing without feeling heavy. Many gel cleansers contain ingredients like salicylic acid, tea tree oil, or niacinamide that provide additional benefits for acne-prone skin.

Cream cleansers have a richer, more nourishing texture that's particularly suitable for dry or sensitive skin. They often contain moisturizing ingredients like glycerin, ceramides, or hyaluronic acid that help maintain hydration while cleansing. Cream cleansers are less likely to cause dryness or irritation, making them ideal for those with compromised skin barriers.

Foam cleansers create a rich lather when mixed with water and are popular for their satisfying, thorough-feeling cleanse. However, many traditional foam cleansers contain sulfates that can be drying and irritating. Asian foam cleansers often use gentler surfactants like coco-glucoside or sodium cocoyl isethionate that provide effective cleansing without stripping the skin.

Low-pH cleansers are specifically formulated to maintain the skin's natural acid mantle. These cleansers typically have a pH between 4.5 and 6.5, which helps preserve the skin's protective barrier and beneficial microbiome. Low-pH cleansers are particularly important for those with sensitive, acne-prone, or compromised skin.

The Importance of pH in Cleansing

The pH level of your cleanser significantly impacts your skin's health and appearance. The skin's natural pH is slightly acidic, with an average of around 5.5. This acidic environment helps maintain the skin's protective barrier, supports beneficial bacteria, and inhibits the growth of harmful microorganisms [22].

Traditional soaps and many cleansers have an alkaline pH of 8-10, which can disrupt the skin's acid mantle and lead to dryness, irritation, and increased susceptibility to environmental damage. Studies have shown that using alkaline cleansers can raise the skin's pH for several hours after cleansing, during which time the skin is more vulnerable to irritation and bacterial overgrowth [23].

Emphasis on low-pH cleansers helps maintain the skin's natural protective mechanisms while still providing effective cleansing. This approach is particularly beneficial for those with sensitive, acne-prone, or aging skin, as maintaining optimal pH supports the skin's natural repair and renewal processes.

Specialized Cleansing Techniques

The 60-Second Rule

This technique involves extending the cleansing time to ensure thorough removal of impurities and provide gentle stimulation that can improve circulation. Spend a full 60 seconds massaging your cleanser into the skin, using gentle circular motions and paying attention to all areas of the face and neck.

The extended massage time allows the cleanser to work more effectively while providing a relaxing, spa-like experience. This technique is particularly beneficial for those who wear makeup regularly or live in polluted environments, as it ensures more complete removal of accumulated impurities.

Konjac Sponge Cleansing

Konjac sponges, made from the root of the konjac plant, provide gentle physical exfoliation while cleansing. These natural sponges become soft and squishy when wet, making them suitable even for sensitive skin. They help remove dead skin cells and improve product absorption while providing a satisfying tactile experience.

To use a konjac sponge, soak it in warm water until it becomes soft, then gently massage it over the face in circular motions with or without cleanser. The sponge provides mild exfoliation that's gentler than traditional scrubs while still helping to improve skin texture and radiance.

Micellar Water Cleansing

Micellar water contains tiny oil molecules called micelles that attract and lift away dirt, oil, and makeup without the need for rinsing. While not a replacement for thorough double cleansing, micellar water can be useful for quick cleansing, removing makeup before oil cleansing, or cleansing when water isn't available.

Asian micellar waters often contain additional beneficial ingredients like hyaluronic acid, ceramides, or botanical extracts that provide skincare benefits beyond cleansing. They're particularly useful for sensitive skin types or when traveling.

Cleansing Balm

Cleansing balms combine the benefits of oil cleansing with the convenience of a solid texture that melts on contact with the skin. These products often contain a blend of oils and waxes that provide effective cleansing while nourishing the skin.

Common Cleansing Mistakes to Avoid

Understanding common cleansing mistakes can help you avoid practices that might be undermining your skincare efforts. One of the most frequent errors is using water that's too hot, which can strip the skin's natural oils and cause irritation. Lukewarm water is ideal for cleansing, as it's effective at removing impurities without being damaging to the skin.

Over-cleansing is another common mistake, particularly among those dealing with acne or oily skin. Cleansing more than twice daily can disrupt the skin barrier and actually worsen the problems you're trying to solve. Stick to morning and evening cleansing, and use appropriate treatments rather than increasing cleansing frequency.

Using the wrong products for your skin type can also undermine your cleansing efforts. A cleanser that works well for your friend may not be appropriate for your skin, so it's important to choose products based on your individual needs rather than recommendations alone.

Rushing the cleansing process reduces its effectiveness and can lead to incomplete removal of impurities. Take the time to cleanse thoroughly, allowing the products to work effectively and enjoying the process as a moment of self-care in your daily routine.

The Role of Cleansing in Overall Skin Health

Proper cleansing does more than just remove dirt and makeup—it plays a crucial role in overall skin health and the effectiveness of your entire skincare routine. Clean skin absorbs subsequent products more effectively, allowing serums, moisturizers, and treatments to penetrate properly and deliver their intended benefits.

Regular, gentle cleansing also supports the skin's natural renewal processes by removing dead skin cells and allowing new, healthy cells to surface. This process helps maintain a smooth, radiant complexion and can improve the appearance of fine lines, uneven texture, and dullness.

The massage aspect of cleansing provides additional benefits by stimulating circulation, which brings nutrients to the skin cells and helps remove waste products. This increased circulation can contribute to a healthy, glowing complexion and may help support the skin's natural repair processes.

Building Your Cleansing Routine

Develop a cleansing routine that suits your skin type, lifestyle, and personal preferences. Start with basic products and adjust based on how your skin responds. Remember that consistency is more important than complexity—a simple routine done consistently will deliver better results than a complex one used sporadically. Pay attention to how your skin feels after cleansing. It should feel clean but not tight, refreshed but not dry. If you experience tightness, dryness, or irritation, adjust your routine by using gentler products or reducing the frequency of cleansing.

Be patient as you find the right products and techniques for your skin. It may take some experimentation to discover what works best, and your needs may change based on factors like season, age, or lifestyle changes. The key is to maintain the principles of gentle, thorough cleansing while adapting the specifics to your individual circumstances.

Remember that cleansing is not just about removing impurities—it's also an opportunity for self-care and mindfulness. Approach your cleansing routine as a moment of calm in your day, taking the time to care for your skin and yourself. This mindful approach to cleansing embodies the philosophy that skincare is not just about achieving beautiful skin, but about creating moments of peace and self-care in our daily lives.

CHAPTER 6:
ESSENCES, TONERS & SERUMS

The Heart of Asian Skincare Innovation

Essences, toners, and serums represent the innovative core of Asian skincare, embodying the philosophy of layered hydration and targeted treatment that has revolutionized global beauty practices. These products serve as the bridge between basic cleansing and moisturizing, delivering concentrated benefits that transform skin health and appearance over time.

The Asian approach to these intermediate steps reflects a sophisticated understanding of skin physiology and the recognition that different molecular sizes and formulation types can address various skin needs simultaneously. Unlike the "one-size-fits-all" approach of traditional moisturizers, this method uses multiple lightweight layers to deliver hydration, active ingredients, and targeted treatments in a way that maximizes absorption and minimizes irritation.

This layering philosophy is supported by extensive research in transdermal drug delivery, which has shown that sequential application of products with different molecular weights and formulation types can enhance penetration and efficacy. The Asian beauty industry has leveraged this scientific understanding to create products that work synergistically, with each layer enhancing the effectiveness of the others.

Understanding Toners: Beyond Astringency

Asian toners represent a fundamental departure from traditional Western astringent toners. While Western toners historically focused on removing residual impurities and tightening pores through alcohol-based formulations, Asian toners prioritize hydration, pH balancing, and skin preparation for subsequent products.

The Science of pH Balancing

The primary function of Asian toners is to restore the skin's optimal pH after cleansing. Even gentle cleansers can temporarily raise the skin's pH, and tap water in many areas is alkaline, further disrupting the skin's natural acid mantle. Asian toners typically have a pH between 4.5 and 6.0, helping to quickly restore the skin's protective acidic environment.

Research has demonstrated that maintaining optimal skin pH is crucial for barrier function, enzyme activity, and microbial balance. A study published in the Journal of Investigative Dermatology found that even small deviations from optimal pH can significantly impact the skin's ability to repair itself and defend against environmental stressors [24]. This scientific understanding validates the emphasis on pH-balancing toners as an essential step in skincare routines.

Hydrating Toner Formulations

Modern Asian toners are formulated with humectants, emollients, and beneficial actives that provide immediate and long-term skin benefits.

Hyaluronic acid, glycerin, and sodium PCA are common humectants that draw moisture to the skin, while ingredients like ceramides, cholesterol, and fatty acids help strengthen the skin barrier.

Many Asian toners also incorporate fermented ingredients, botanical extracts, and gentle acids that provide additional benefits beyond hydration. These formulations are designed to be layered, with the famous "7-skin method" involving multiple applications of toner to achieve intense hydration and plumping effects.

The Essence Revolution: Fermentation and Innovation

Essences represent one of Asia's most significant contributions to global skincare, introducing the concept of lightweight, highly concentrated treatments that bridge the gap between toners and serums. These products typically contain higher concentrations of active ingredients than toners but are lighter and more easily absorbed than traditional serums.

Fermented Ingredients: The Asian Advantage

Asian skincare has pioneered the use of fermented ingredients in cosmetic formulations, leveraging traditional fermentation techniques to enhance the bioavailability and effectiveness of natural ingredients. Fermentation breaks down large molecules into smaller, more easily absorbed components while creating beneficial byproducts that can improve skin health.

Galactomyces ferment filtrate, one of the most popular fermented ingredients in essences, is produced by fermenting yeast in a controlled environment. Research has shown that this ingredient can improve skin hydration, reduce hyperpigmentation, and provide antioxidant benefits.

The fermentation process creates amino acids, vitamins, and organic acids that are more bioavailable than their non-fermented counterparts.

Bifida ferment lysate, another popular fermented ingredient, is derived from beneficial bacteria and has been shown to strengthen the skin barrier, improve hydration, and enhance the skin's natural repair processes. Studies have demonstrated that this ingredient can help protect against environmental stressors and support healthy skin microbiome balance [25].

Serums: Targeted Treatment Powerhouses

Serums represent the most concentrated form of active ingredients in Asian skincare routines, designed to address specific skin concerns with precision and efficacy. These products typically contain 10-20% active ingredients, compared to 1-5% in moisturizers, making them powerful tools for addressing issues like hyperpigmentation, aging, acne, and dehydration.

Niacinamide: The Multi-Functional Marvel

Niacinamide, also known as nicotinamide or vitamin B3, has become one of the most popular and well-researched ingredients in Asian serums. This water-soluble vitamin provides multiple benefits including pore refinement, oil control, brightening, and anti-inflammatory effects, making it suitable for virtually all skin types and concerns.

The mechanism of action for niacinamide involves its role as a precursor to NAD+ (nicotinamide adenine dinucleotide), a coenzyme essential for cellular energy production and DNA repair. Research has shown that topical niacinamide can improve skin barrier function, reduce transepidermal water loss, and enhance the skin's natural repair processes [26].

Clinical studies have demonstrated that niacinamide concentrations of 2-5% can significantly improve skin texture, reduce hyperpigmentation, and minimize the appearance of pores. Higher concentrations (up to 10%) may provide additional benefits but can also increase the risk of irritation, particularly for sensitive skin types.

Vitamin C: Antioxidant Protection and Brightening

Vitamin C serums are among the most popular and effective treatments for brightening, antioxidant protection, and anti-aging. However, vitamin C is notoriously unstable and can degrade quickly when exposed to light, air, or heat. Asian formulations have addressed these challenges through innovative stabilization techniques and derivative forms that maintain efficacy while improving stability.

L-ascorbic acid is the most potent form of vitamin C but also the most unstable. Asian serums often use stabilized derivatives like magnesium ascorbyl phosphate, sodium ascorbyl phosphate, or ascorbyl glucoside that provide similar benefits with improved stability and reduced irritation potential.

The antioxidant properties of vitamin C help protect against environmental damage, while its role in collagen synthesis supports skin firmness and elasticity. Vitamin C also inhibits tyrosinase, the enzyme responsible for melanin production, making it effective for preventing and fading hyperpigmentation.

Peptides: The Anti-Aging Innovators

Peptides are short chains of amino acids that can signal the skin to perform specific functions, such as producing collagen, reducing inflammation, or improving barrier function. Asian serums often feature innovative peptide complexes that target multiple signs of aging simultaneously.

Copper peptides, such as copper tripeptide-1, have been shown to stimulate collagen production and improve skin firmness. Palmitoyl pentapeptide-4 (Matrixyl) can reduce the appearance of fine lines and wrinkles by promoting collagen synthesis. Acetyl hexapeptide-8 (Argireline) provides a botox-like effect by reducing muscle contractions that contribute to expression lines.

The effectiveness of peptides depends on their ability to penetrate the skin and reach their target cells. Asian formulations often use advanced delivery systems and penetration enhancers to improve peptide absorption and efficacy. However, these serums often require gradual introduction to build tolerance.

Product Recommendations by Skin Type and Concern

For Oily and Acne-Prone Skin

Niacinamide serums at 2-5% concentration can help control oil production and minimize pores. Look for lightweight, gel-based formulations that won't clog pores. Tea tree oil or salicylic acid can provide additional acne-fighting benefits.

Hydrating essences with fermented ingredients like galactomyces can provide necessary moisture without adding oil. Avoid heavy, occlusive formulations that might clog pores.

For Dry and Sensitive Skin

Hyaluronic acid serums with multiple molecular weights provide intense hydration without irritation. Look for formulations with additional barrier-supporting ingredients like ceramides or cholesterol.

Gentle essences with fermented ingredients or botanical extracts can provide hydration and soothing benefits. Avoid products with high concentrations of acids or alcohol that might cause irritation.

For Aging and Mature Skin

Peptide serums can help stimulate collagen production and improve skin firmness. Look for formulations that combine multiple peptides for comprehensive anti-aging benefits.

Vitamin C serums provide antioxidant protection and can help improve skin brightness and texture. Choose stabilized forms if you have sensitive skin or are new to vitamin C.

For Hyperpigmentation and Uneven Tone

Niacinamide serums can help prevent and fade dark spots while improving overall skin texture. Arbutin, kojic acid, or licorice root extract can provide additional brightening benefits.

Vitamin C serums are excellent for preventing new pigmentation and gradually fading existing spots. Consistent use over 3-6 months typically shows significant results.

The Future of Essence and Serum Innovation

Asian skincare continues to push the boundaries of innovation in essence and serum formulations. Emerging trends include personalized formulations based on genetic testing, microbiome-supporting ingredients, and advanced delivery systems that enhance ingredient penetration and efficacy.

Fermentation technology continues to evolve, with new strains of beneficial bacteria and yeast being explored for their skincare benefits. Postbiotic ingredients, which are the beneficial byproducts of probiotic fermentation, are gaining attention for their ability to support skin health without the stability concerns of live probiotics.

Nanotechnology and encapsulation techniques are being used to improve the stability and delivery of active ingredients, allowing for more potent formulations with reduced irritation potential. These advances promise to make effective skincare more accessible and suitable for a wider range of skin types and concerns.

The Asian approach to essences, toners, and serums represents a sophisticated understanding of skin physiology and the power of layered, targeted treatments. By incorporating these products into your routine and understanding how to use them effectively, you can achieve the hydrated, healthy, radiant skin that Asian skincare is famous for promoting. The key is patience, consistency, and a willingness to listen to your skin's needs as they change over time.

CHAPTER 7: HYDRATION & BARRIER REPAIR:

Hyaluronic Acid, Ceramides & Ferments

The Science of Skin Hydration

Hydration forms the cornerstone of Asian skincare philosophy, reflecting a deep understanding that well-hydrated skin is not only more beautiful but also more resilient, functional, and capable of self-repair. The Asian approach to hydration goes far beyond simply applying moisturizer, encompassing a sophisticated understanding of how water moves through the skin, what factors influence moisture retention, and how different ingredients work synergistically to maintain optimal hydration levels [27].

The skin's hydration system is remarkably complex, involving multiple layers, cellular structures, and biochemical processes that work together to maintain moisture balance. The stratum corneum, the outermost layer of the epidermis, acts as both a protective barrier and a reservoir for water, containing approximately 10-30% water under normal conditions. When this water content drops below 10%, the skin becomes dry, flaky, and compromised in its protective function [28].

Asian skincare's multi-layered approach to hydration recognizes that different types of moisture-binding ingredients work at different levels of the skin and through different mechanisms. This understanding has led to the development of sophisticated formulations that combine humectants, emollients, and occlusives in precise ratios to provide both immediate and long-lasting hydration benefits.

Understanding the Skin Barrier

The skin barrier, also known as the stratum corneum or acid mantle, represents one of the body's most important protective systems. This thin but crucial layer consists of corneocytes (dead skin cells) embedded in a lipid matrix, often compared to a brick-and-mortar structure where the cells are bricks and the lipids are mortar. This structure provides protection against environmental stressors while preventing excessive water loss.

The Lipid Matrix Composition

The lipid matrix that holds the skin barrier together consists primarily of three types of lipids: ceramides (approximately 50%), cholesterol (25%), and free fatty acids (15-25%). These lipids are arranged in highly organized bilayer structures that create an effective barrier against water loss while allowing the passage of certain beneficial substances [29].

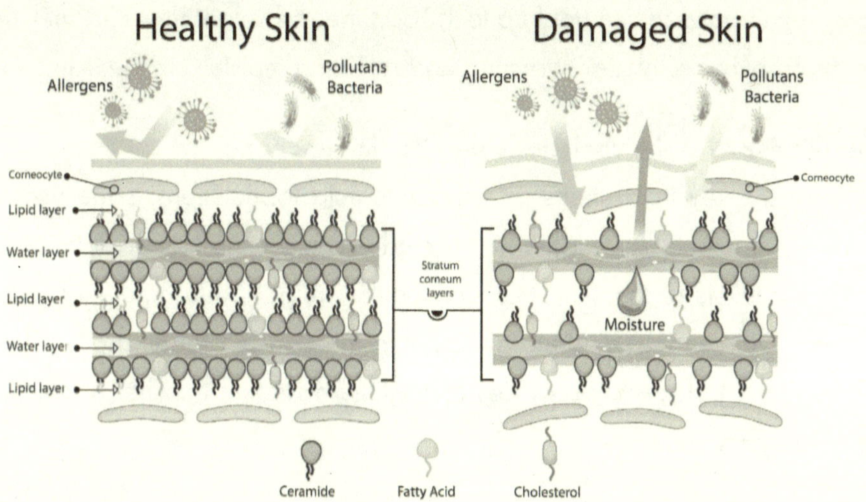

Ceramides are perhaps the most important component of the barrier lipids, serving as both structural elements and signaling molecules that regulate barrier function. There are at least nine different types of ceramides in human skin, each with specific functions and characteristics. Asian skincare has been at the forefront of incorporating various ceramide types into formulations to support and restore barrier function [30].

Cholesterol plays a crucial role in maintaining the fluidity and permeability of the lipid bilayers, while free fatty acids help maintain the skin's acidic pH and provide antimicrobial protection. The precise ratio and organization of these lipids are essential for optimal barrier function, and disruption of this balance can lead to increased water loss, sensitivity, and various skin conditions.

Hyaluronic Acid: The Ultimate Hydrator

Hyaluronic acid has become synonymous with hydration in Asian skincare, and scientific research validates its reputation as one of the most effective moisturizing ingredients available. This naturally occurring glycosaminoglycan can hold up to 1,000 times its weight in water, making it incredibly effective for attracting and retaining moisture in the skin.

Molecular Weight Variations and Their Functions

One of the key innovations in hyaluronic acid formulations is the use of multiple molecular weights to provide comprehensive hydration at different levels of the skin. High molecular weight hyaluronic acid (over 1,000 kDa) cannot penetrate deeply into the skin but forms a protective film on the surface that provides immediate hydration and helps prevent moisture loss.

Medium molecular weight hyaluronic acid (50-1,000 kDa) can penetrate into the upper layers of the epidermis, providing sustained hydration and plumping effects. Low molecular weight hyaluronic acid (under 50 kDa) can penetrate deeper into the skin, providing long-lasting hydration and supporting the skin's natural moisture-retention mechanisms.

Asian skincare formulations often combine all three molecular weights to create a multi-layered hydration effect that addresses both immediate and long-term moisture needs. This approach is particularly beneficial for dehydrated skin, aging skin, and those living in challenging climatic conditions [31].

Sodium Hyaluronate vs. Hyaluronic Acid

Sodium hyaluronate, the sodium salt of hyaluronic acid, is often used in skincare formulations because it's more stable and has better penetration properties than pure hyaluronic acid. The smaller molecular size of sodium hyaluronate allows it to penetrate more easily into the skin, where it can attract and bind water more effectively.

Asian formulations often use both hyaluronic acid and sodium hyaluronate in combination, leveraging the surface hydration benefits of hyaluronic acid with the deeper penetration and longer-lasting effects of sodium hyaluronate. This combination provides comprehensive hydration that works both immediately and over time.

Ceramides: The Barrier Builders

Ceramides represent one of the most important innovations in modern skincare, offering the ability to directly replenish and restore the skin's natural barrier function. These lipid molecules are identical to those found naturally in the skin, making them highly compatible and effective for barrier repair and maintenance [32].

Types of Ceramides and Their Functions

Human skin contains at least nine different types of ceramides, each with specific functions and characteristics. Ceramide 1 (now called Ceramide EOS) is crucial for barrier function and is often deficient in conditions like atopic dermatitis. Ceramide 3 (Ceramide NP) is the most abundant ceramide in healthy skin and plays a key role in maintaining barrier integrity.

It's important for skincare formulations to include multiple ceramide types to provide comprehensive barrier support. Ceramide AP helps maintain skin smoothness and flexibility, while Ceramide NS supports barrier function and helps prevent moisture loss. The combination of different ceramides can provide more effective barrier repair than single ceramide formulations.

Phytoceramides, derived from plants, offer similar benefits to human ceramides while being more stable and cost-effective to produce. These plant-derived ceramides can help restore barrier function and improve hydration, though they may be slightly less effective than identical human ceramides.

Ceramide Delivery and Formulation Challenges

Ceramides are challenging to formulate because they're naturally solid at room temperature and can be difficult to incorporate into stable, cosmetically elegant products. Modern formulations have developed sophisticated delivery systems that maintain ceramide stability while ensuring effective penetration into the skin [33].

Liposomal delivery systems encapsulate ceramides in lipid vesicles that can fuse with the skin's natural lipid layers, delivering ceramides directly where they're needed. Nano-emulsion technology creates extremely small particles that can penetrate more effectively while maintaining product stability.

The ratio of ceramides to other barrier lipids is crucial for effectiveness. Asian formulations often include cholesterol and fatty acids in ratios that mimic the natural composition of healthy skin barriers, providing comprehensive barrier support rather than just ceramide supplementation.

Clinical Evidence for Ceramide Effectiveness

Extensive clinical research has demonstrated the effectiveness of topical ceramides for improving barrier function, reducing water loss, and alleviating various skin conditions. Studies have shown that ceramide-containing moisturizers can significantly improve skin hydration, reduce irritation, and help restore normal barrier function in compromised skin [34].

Research specifically focused on ceramide formulations has shown that products containing multiple ceramide types with appropriate delivery systems can provide superior barrier repair compared to single-ingredient or poorly formulated products. These studies validate the approach of using multi-component formulations for optimal skin benefits [35].

Climate Adaptation: Hydration Strategies for Different Environments

Understanding how environmental factors affect skin hydration allows for more effective product selection and application techniques that optimize results regardless of location or season.

Humid Climate Considerations

In humid environments, the skin's natural moisture retention mechanisms work more effectively, and lighter hydration formulations may be sufficient. However, high humidity can also increase the risk of bacterial growth and may require adjustments to prevent clogged pores or breakouts.

Strategies for humid climates focus on lightweight, fast-absorbing formulations that provide adequate moisture without feeling heavy or greasy. Gel-based moisturizers, lightweight essences, and water-based serums are particularly effective in these conditions.

The layering technique becomes even more important in humid climates, as multiple thin layers can provide adequate hydration without the heaviness that might feel uncomfortable in high humidity.

Dry Climate Adaptations

Dry climates present significant challenges for skin hydration, as low humidity levels can rapidly draw moisture from the skin, leading to dehydration, irritation, and barrier compromise. Asian hydration strategies for dry climates emphasize occlusive ingredients and barrier support to prevent moisture loss.

In dry environments, the routine may include additional hydrating layers, richer moisturizers, and more frequent application of hydrating products. Facial oils, sleeping masks, and occlusive treatments become particularly important for maintaining adequate hydration levels.

The timing of product application also becomes crucial in dry climates. Applying hydrating products immediately after cleansing, while the skin is still damp, helps trap moisture and enhance the effectiveness of subsequent products. Humidifiers and other environmental modifications can also support skincare efforts in very dry conditions.

Seasonal Transitions and Adaptation

Skin hydration needs change significantly with the seasons. Winter typically requires richer, more occlusive formulations to combat dry air and indoor heating, while summer may call for lighter, more breathable products.

Spring and fall transitions can be particularly challenging for skin hydration, as rapid changes in temperature and humidity can disrupt the skin's natural adaptation mechanisms. During these periods, use gentle, barrier-supporting products that help the skin adjust to changing conditions without becoming irritated or compromised.

For seasonal adaptation it's better to gradually transition between different product formulations rather than making sudden changes that might shock the skin. This gradual approach allows the skin to adapt while maintaining optimal hydration and barrier function throughout the year.

Hydration Techniques

The 7-Skin Method

The 7-skin method, involving multiple applications of hydrating toner, represents one of Asia's most innovative contributions to hydration techniques. This method is based on the principle that multiple thin layers can provide more effective hydration than a single thick application while also providing a meditative, self-care experience.

Scientific studies support this approach, showing that multiple applications of hydrating products can significantly increase skin moisture levels and improve barrier function. The technique is particularly beneficial for dehydrated skin, aging skin, and those living in dry climates.

The 7-skin method can be adapted based on individual needs and environmental conditions. In humid climates or for oily skin, 3-5 layers may be sufficient, while dry climates or very dehydrated skin may benefit from the full seven layers. The key is listening to your skin and adjusting accordingly.

Hydrating Sheet Masks

Sheet masks have revolutionized the delivery of intensive hydration treatments, providing a convenient and effective way to deliver high concentrations of hydrating ingredients. The occlusive effect of the mask material enhances ingredient penetration while preventing evaporation.

Hydrating sheet masks typically contain combinations of hyaluronic acid, ceramides, and fermented ingredients in concentrations higher than those found in regular skincare products. The 15-20 minute application time allows for maximum absorption while providing a relaxing, spa-like experience.

For optimal results, sheet masks should be used on clean skin and followed with a moisturizer to seal in the benefits. The frequency of use can be adjusted based on skin needs, with some people using masks daily while others find 2-3 times per week sufficient.

Sleeping Masks and Overnight Treatments

Sleeping masks represent another innovation in hydration delivery, providing intensive overnight treatment that works with the skin's natural repair processes. These products are typically more occlusive than regular moisturizers, creating a protective barrier that prevents moisture loss while delivering active ingredients.

The skin's repair and regeneration processes are most active during sleep, making overnight treatments particularly effective for hydration and barrier repair. Sleeping masks often contain time-release ingredients that provide sustained benefits throughout the night.

Asian sleeping masks frequently combine multiple hydrating ingredients with barrier-supporting lipids and antioxidants to provide comprehensive overnight skin treatment. These products are designed to be left on overnight and either absorbed completely or gently removed in the morning.

Product Recommendations for Different Skin Types

For Oily and Combination Skin

Oily skin still requires adequate hydration, but benefits from lightweight, non-comedogenic formulations that won't clog pores or feel heavy. Gel-based moisturizers with hyaluronic acid, lightweight essences with fermented ingredients, and water-based serums are ideal for providing hydration without adding excess oil [36].

Niacinamide is particularly beneficial for oily skin, as it helps regulate sebum production while providing hydration and barrier support. Combination skin may require different products for different areas of the face, with lighter formulations for the T-zone and richer products for drier areas.

For Dry and Sensitive Skin

Dry and sensitive skin requires gentle, nourishing formulations that provide intense hydration while supporting barrier repair. Cream-based moisturizers with ceramides, essences with fermented ingredients, and facial oils can provide the rich hydration that dry skin needs [37].

Sensitive skin benefits from minimal, fragrance-free formulations with proven hydrating ingredients. Hyaluronic acid, ceramides, and gentle fermented ingredients are typically well-tolerated and effective for sensitive skin types.

For Aging and Mature Skin

Aging skin often has compromised barrier function and reduced natural moisture production, requiring intensive hydration and barrier support. Multi-molecular weight hyaluronic acid, ceramide-rich moisturizers, and peptide-containing treatments can help address the specific needs of mature skin.

Antioxidant-rich formulations that combine hydration with anti-aging benefits are particularly valuable for mature skin. Ingredients like vitamin

C, niacinamide, and fermented extracts can provide both hydration and anti-aging benefits.

The Future of Hydration Science

The skincare industry continues to innovate in hydration technology, with emerging developments including personalized hydration based on genetic testing, advanced delivery systems that enhance ingredient penetration, and new fermentation techniques that create novel hydrating compounds.

Nanotechnology is being used to create more effective delivery systems for hydrating ingredients, while biotechnology is enabling the production of identical human ceramides and other barrier lipids. These advances promise to make effective hydration more accessible and suitable for a wider range of skin types and environmental conditions.

By combining multiple hydrating ingredients with appropriate delivery systems and application techniques, it's possible to achieve and maintain optimal skin hydration regardless of skin type, age, or environmental conditions. The key is understanding your skin's specific needs and adapting your routine accordingly while maintaining consistent and gentle care.

CHAPTER 8:
LAYERING:
The Multi-Step Routine from Cleansing to Sunscreen

The Science of Skincare Layering

The multi-step skincare routine has become popular in the beauty world, but its effectiveness stems from solid scientific principles rather than marketing hype. The layering technique is based on the fundamental principle of applying products from thinnest to thickest consistency, allowing each layer to penetrate effectively before the next is applied. This method maximizes the absorption and effectiveness of active ingredients while minimizing the risk of pilling or reduced efficacy.

The science behind layering lies in understanding how different molecular sizes and formulation types interact with the skin. Water-based products with smaller molecules can penetrate more easily when applied first, while oil-based products with larger molecules form a protective layer that can enhance the absorption of previously applied products. This synergistic effect means that properly layered products often work better together than they would individually.

Research in transdermal drug delivery has shown that the sequential application of products can enhance penetration through various mechanisms. The first layer can act as a penetration enhancer for subsequent layers, while later layers can provide occlusion that drives earlier layers deeper into the skin. This scientific understanding validates the approach to layering and explains why the multi-step routine can be more effective than using fewer, more concentrated products [38].

The Complete Multi-Step Breakdown

The traditional Asian skincare routine can include up to 12 steps, though most modern practitioners use between 7 and 10 steps depending on their skin's needs and time constraints. Each step serves a specific purpose and builds upon the previous one to create a comprehensive approach to skin health and beauty. We have talked about all of these steps previously and their science, now let's go through them in sequence to build a complete skincare routine.

Step 1: Oil Cleanser (Evening Only)

The first step in the evening routine is oil cleansing, which removes makeup, sunscreen, and oil-based impurities that water-based cleansers cannot effectively eliminate. Modern oil cleansers are sophisticated formulations that emulsify when mixed with water, making them easy to rinse off without leaving a greasy residue. Look for cleansing oils that contain emulsifiers like PEG-20 glyceryl triisostearate or polysorbate 80, which ensure complete removal while maintaining the cleansing benefits of oil.

The oil cleansing process should be thorough but gentle. Apply the oil cleanser to dry skin and massage for 1-2 minutes, paying particular attention to areas where makeup or sunscreen accumulates. Add a small amount of water to emulsify the oil, then rinse thoroughly with lukewarm water. This step is crucial for preparing the skin for the water-based cleanser that follows.

Step 2: Water-Based Cleanser

The second cleansing step uses a water-based cleanser to remove any remaining impurities, including sweat, dirt, and water-based products. This step also removes any residue from the oil cleanser, ensuring that the skin is completely clean and ready to absorb subsequent products effectively.

Choose a water-based cleanser with a pH between 4.5 and 6.5 to maintain the skin's natural acid mantle. Ingredients like glycerin, hyaluronic acid, or amino acids provide additional hydration benefits, while avoiding sulfates helps prevent irritation and over-drying. The cleanser should leave your skin feeling clean but not tight or stripped.

Apply the water-based cleanser to damp skin and massage gently for 30-60 seconds. Focus on areas that tend to accumulate oil or impurities, but avoid aggressive scrubbing that can damage the skin barrier. Rinse thoroughly with lukewarm water and gently pat dry with a clean towel.

Step 3: Exfoliation (2-3 Times Per Week)

Exfoliation removes dead skin cells that can clog pores and interfere with product absorption. Asian skincare typically favors chemical exfoliation over physical scrubs, as chemical exfoliants provide more even and gentle exfoliation without the risk of micro-tears that can occur with abrasive scrubs.

Alpha hydroxy acids (AHAs) like glycolic acid and lactic acid work on the skin's surface to remove dead cells and improve texture. Beta hydroxy acids (BHAs) like salicylic acid can penetrate into pores to remove oil and debris. Polyhydroxy acids (PHAs) like gluconolactone provide gentle exfoliation suitable for sensitive skin. Start with lower concentrations and gradually increase as your skin builds tolerance.

Apply exfoliating products to clean, dry skin and allow them to work for the recommended time before proceeding with the rest of your routine. Always follow exfoliation with adequate sun protection, as exfoliated skin is more sensitive to UV damage.

Step 4: Toner

Different from traditional astringent toners. Asian toners are hydrating, pH-balancing products that prepare the skin for better absorption of subsequent products. They often contain beneficial ingredients like hyaluronic acid, glycerin, or botanical extracts that provide additional skincare benefits.

The primary function of an Asian toner is to restore the skin's optimal pH after cleansing and provide the first layer of hydration. This step is particularly important if you use a cleanser with a higher pH or if your tap water is hard or alkaline. Toners also help remove any final traces of cleanser or impurities that might remain on the skin.

Apply toner using the "7-skin method" for maximum hydration benefits. This technique involves applying multiple thin layers of toner, patting each layer into the skin until absorbed before applying the next. This method can provide intense hydration and is particularly beneficial for dry or dehydrated skin.

Step 5: Essence

Essences are lightweight, watery products that contain higher concentrations of active ingredients than toners but are less concentrated than serums. They provide an additional layer of hydration while delivering beneficial ingredients like fermented extracts, peptides, or antioxidants to the skin.

Fermented essences are particularly popular in Asian skincare, as the fermentation process breaks down ingredients into smaller molecules that can penetrate more easily. Ingredients like galactomyces ferment filtrate, bifida ferment lysate, or sake filtrate provide gentle exfoliation, hydration, and antioxidant benefits.

Apply essence by patting it gently into the skin with your palms or fingertips. The patting motion helps stimulate circulation and ensures even distribution. Allow the essence to absorb completely before proceeding to the next step.

Step 6: Treatments/Serums

Serums and treatment products contain the highest concentrations of active ingredients and are designed to address specific skin concerns. This is where you would apply products containing ingredients like vitamin C, niacinamide, retinol, or peptides. The key is to choose treatments that address your primary skin concerns without overwhelming the skin.

When using multiple serums, apply them in order of consistency (thinnest to thickest) and allow each to absorb before applying the next. If using potentially irritating ingredients like retinol or high-concentration acids, start slowly and build tolerance gradually. Some active ingredients should not be used together, so research compatibility before combining treatments.

The "sandwich method" can be useful for applying potent treatments. Apply a thin layer of hydrating essence or toner, then the treatment product, followed by another layer of essence or a hydrating serum. This technique helps buffer potentially irritating ingredients while maintaining their effectiveness.

Step 7: Sheet Masks (2-3 Times Per Week)

Sheet masks provide intensive treatment and hydration in a convenient, mess-free format. They create an occlusive environment that enhances the penetration of active ingredients while providing a relaxing, spa-like experience. There are now countless varieties targeting different skin concerns.

Choose sheet masks based on your current skin needs rather than your skin type. Hydrating masks with hyaluronic acid or ceramides benefit all skin types, while brightening masks with vitamin C or niacinamide can help address hyperpigmentation. Avoid masks with high concentrations of acids or potentially irritating ingredients if you have sensitive skin.

Apply sheet masks to clean skin and leave on for 15-20 minutes. Remove the mask and gently pat any remaining essence into the skin. Don't rinse after using a sheet mask unless the instructions specifically recommend it, as this removes the beneficial ingredients you've just applied.

Step 8: Eye Cream

The delicate eye area has thinner skin and fewer oil glands than the rest of the face, making it more prone to dryness, fine lines, and sensitivity. Eye creams are specially formulated to address these unique needs with gentler, more hydrating formulations.

Look for eye creams with ingredients like peptides for firming, caffeine for reducing puffiness, vitamin C for brightening, or retinol for anti-aging (though retinol should be introduced gradually and may not be suitable for very sensitive eyes). Avoid products with strong fragrances or essential oils that might irritate the sensitive eye area.

Apply eye cream using your ring finger, which applies the least pressure. Gently pat the product around the orbital bone, avoiding the immediate eye area and being careful not to pull or stretch the delicate skin.

Step 9: Moisturizer/Cream

Moisturizer provides essential hydration and helps seal in all the previous layers of products. Asian moisturizers often have lighter textures, focusing on hydration rather than heavy occlusion. Choose a moisturizer appropriate for your skin type and the current season.

For oily skin, look for gel-based or lightweight lotion moisturizers with ingredients like hyaluronic acid or niacinamide. Dry skin benefits from cream-based moisturizers with ceramides, cholesterol, or fatty acids. Combination skin may require different moisturizers for different areas of the face.

Apply moisturizer using upward strokes, starting from the center of the face and working outward. Don't forget often-neglected areas like the neck, ears, and around the hairline. Allow the moisturizer to absorb completely before applying sunscreen or makeup.

Step 10: Sunscreen (Morning Only)

Sunscreen is the most important step in any morning skincare routine, as UV exposure is the primary cause of premature aging and skin damage. Asian sunscreens are renowned for their elegant textures, high protection levels, and additional skincare benefits that make daily application more pleasant.

Choose a broad-spectrum sunscreen with at least SPF 30, though SPF 50+ is preferable for extended outdoor exposure. Asian sunscreens often incorporate skincare ingredients like hyaluronic acid, niacinamide, or antioxidants, providing additional benefits beyond UV protection.

Apply sunscreen generously—most people use only 25-50% of the recommended amount. Use approximately 1/4 teaspoon (or 1.25ml) for the face and neck, and reapply every 2 hours or after swimming, sweating, or toweling off. If you are not sure how much sunscreen is 1/4 teaspoon, use the "nickel sized dollop" rule or the "2 finger rule". Don't forget often-missed areas like the ears, neck, and around the eyes.

Additional Optional Steps

Cleansing Mask (1-2 Times Per Week, DO NOT use on same day as exfoliation)

Cleansing masks provide deep purification beyond what daily cleansers can achieve, making them an excellent addition to the enhanced routine. These specialized treatments can be clay-based for oil control, charcoal-based for deep pore cleansing, or enzyme-based for gentle exfoliation and brightening.

Clay masks containing bentonite, kaolin, or French green clay are particularly effective for oily and combination skin types. These clays have a negative charge that attracts positively charged impurities, toxins, and excess oil from the pores. The absorption properties of clay also help to temporarily tighten pores and create a smoother skin texture.

Charcoal masks utilize activated charcoal's porous structure to draw out impurities from deep within the pores. The large surface area of activated charcoal allows it to bind to bacteria, toxins, and excess oil, making it particularly beneficial for acne-prone skin or those exposed to high levels of environmental pollution.

Enzyme masks containing papain from papaya, bromelain from pineapple, or pumpkin enzymes provide gentle chemical exfoliation while deep cleansing. These natural enzymes break down the proteins that hold dead skin cells together, revealing brighter, smoother skin underneath while simultaneously removing impurities.

Apply cleansing masks to clean, dry skin, avoiding the delicate eye area. Follow the manufacturer's instructions for timing, typically 10-15 minutes for clay masks and 5-10 minutes for enzyme masks. Remove with lukewarm water using gentle circular motions, then follow with your regular routine. Use cleansing masks 1-2 times per week, adjusting frequency based on your skin's response and needs.

Moisturizing Mist (Can be Used at Any Time, Particularly for Dry Environment)

Moisturizing mists provide an additional layer of hydration and can deliver beneficial ingredients in a fine, even application that doesn't disturb previous layers. These lightweight formulations can contain thermal spring water, botanical extracts, hyaluronic acid, or other hydrating and soothing ingredients.

The science behind facial mists lies in their ability to provide immediate hydration to the skin's surface while creating a humid microenvironment that can enhance the absorption of subsequent products. Thermal spring water mists, in particular, contain naturally occurring minerals like selenium, silica, and bicarbonates that have anti-inflammatory and antioxidant properties.

Hydrating mists containing hyaluronic acid or glycerin can hold up to 1000 times their weight in water, providing intense hydration that plumps the skin and creates an optimal environment for the absorption of serums and treatments that follow. Some mists also contain peptides, antioxidants, or botanical extracts that provide additional skincare benefits.

Apply facial mist by holding the bottle 6-8 inches away from your face and spraying in a fine, even layer. Allow the mist to settle for 10-15 seconds, then gently pat any excess into the skin with your palms. This step is particularly beneficial for those with dehydrated skin, those living in dry climates, or during air travel when cabin pressure can dehydrate the skin.

Facial mists can also be used throughout the day over makeup to refresh and hydrate the skin, making them a versatile addition to your skincare arsenal. Choose alcohol-free formulations to avoid drying effects, and look for mists in UV-protective packaging to preserve the stability of active ingredients.

Facial Oil (Evening Only)

Facial oils provide an additional layer of nourishment and can help seal in all the previous layers of hydration and treatment products. They contain essential fatty acids, antioxidants, and other beneficial compounds that support skin barrier function and provide anti-aging benefits.

Different oils offer different benefits: rosehip oil is rich in vitamin C and essential fatty acids for anti-aging and brightening; jojoba oil closely mimics the skin's natural sebum and is suitable for all skin types; argan oil contains vitamin E and essential fatty acids for hydration and protection; squalane is lightweight and non-comedogenic, making it suitable for oily skin types.

Apply 2-3 drops of facial oil to your palms, warm between your hands, and gently press into the skin. Focus on areas that tend to be drier, such as the cheeks and around the eyes. Facial oils should be used in the evening routine only, as they can interfere with sunscreen application and effectiveness.

Gua-Sha/Jade Rolling (Evening Only, 1-3 Times Per Week)

Gua-sha and jade rolling are ancient Chinese facial massage techniques that have gained popularity in modern skincare routines for their ability to promote lymphatic drainage, improve circulation, and enhance product absorption. These tools provide a therapeutic massage that can help reduce puffiness, improve skin tone, and create a more sculpted facial appearance while offering a relaxing, meditative experience.

The science behind facial massage tools lies in their ability to stimulate the lymphatic system, which is responsible for removing toxins and excess fluid from tissues. The gentle pressure and specific movements used in gua-sha and jade rolling help move lymphatic fluid toward drainage points, reducing puffiness and promoting a more defined facial contour. Additionally, the massage action increases blood circulation, bringing oxygen and nutrients to the skin cells while promoting the natural healing process.

Gua-sha tools are typically made from smooth stones like jade, rose quartz, or stainless steel, and feature various edges and curves designed to work with the natural contours of the face. The technique involves using gentle pressure and specific strokes to massage the face, following the natural lymphatic drainage pathways. Jade rollers consist of two smooth stone rollers of different sizes mounted on a handle, with the larger roller used for broader areas like the cheeks and forehead, and the smaller roller designed for delicate areas around the eyes.

The benefits of regular facial massage with these tools extend beyond immediate aesthetic improvements. Studies have shown that facial massage can increase blood flow by up to 25%, which enhances the delivery of nutrients to skin cells and promotes collagen production. The mechanical stimulation also helps improve muscle tone in the facial muscles, which can contribute to a more lifted and youthful appearance over time.

When incorporating gua-sha or jade rolling into your routine, timing is crucial for maximum effectiveness. These techniques work best when the skin has a layer of oil or serum to provide adequate slip and prevent dragging or irritation. This makes the placement after facial oil application ideal, as the oil provides the perfect medium for smooth tool movement while the massage helps drive the beneficial ingredients deeper into the skin.

For gua-sha technique, begin with clean tools and clean hands. Start at the center of the face and work outward, using gentle but firm pressure. Begin with the forehead, using upward and outward strokes from the center toward the temples. Move to the eye area, using the curved edge of the tool to gently massage from the inner corner of the eye outward toward the temple, being careful to use very light pressure in this delicate area.

For the cheeks, use long, sweeping strokes from the nose toward the ears, following the natural contours of the face. Work on the jawline using upward strokes from the center of the chin toward the ears, which helps promote lymphatic drainage and can improve the appearance of jaw definition. Finish with the neck, using downward strokes from the jawline toward the collarbone to encourage lymphatic drainage.

Jade rolling technique is somewhat simpler but equally effective. Begin with the larger roller on the forehead, rolling from the center outward toward the temples. Use the smaller roller around the delicate eye area, rolling gently from the inner corner outward. For the cheeks, roll from the nose toward the ears, and use upward rolling motions along the jawline from the chin toward the ears.

The pressure used should be firm enough to feel effective but gentle enough to avoid causing redness or irritation. The goal is to stimulate circulation and lymphatic flow without damaging the delicate facial tissues. Each area should be massaged for 30-60 seconds, with the entire routine taking 5-10 minutes.

Tool maintenance is important for both hygiene and effectiveness. Clean your gua-sha tool or jade roller after each use with gentle soap and warm water, then dry thoroughly. Some practitioners prefer to store their tools in the refrigerator, as the cool temperature can provide additional benefits for reducing puffiness and creating a refreshing sensation during use.

The frequency of gua-sha or jade rolling can be adjusted based on your skin's response and your personal preferences. Most people benefit from using these techniques 3-4 times per week, though daily use is generally safe for most skin types. Those with very sensitive skin or active breakouts should use these tools less frequently and with lighter pressure.

It's important to note that while gua-sha and jade rolling can provide immediate improvements in skin appearance, particularly in terms of reduced puffiness and improved glow, the long-term benefits come from consistent use over time. Like any skincare practice, patience and consistency are key to seeing lasting results.

Sleeping Pack (Evening Only, 1-3 Times Per Week)

Sleeping packs, also known as overnight masks, are intensive treatment products designed to work while you sleep. These occlusive formulations create a protective barrier that prevents transepidermal water loss while delivering high concentrations of beneficial ingredients throughout the night.

The science behind sleeping packs lies in their ability to create an optimal healing environment for the skin during the body's natural repair cycle. During sleep, skin cell regeneration increases, blood flow to the skin improves, and the skin's permeability increases, making it more receptive to active ingredients.

Sleeping packs can be hydrating, anti-aging, brightening, or purifying, depending on their formulation. Hydrating sleeping packs often contain hyaluronic acid, ceramides, or botanical extracts that provide intense moisture. Anti-aging sleeping packs may contain peptides, retinol, or antioxidants that work to repair and prevent signs of aging. Brightening sleeping packs typically include vitamin C, niacinamide, or botanical extracts that help even skin tone and reduce hyperpigmentation.

Apply sleeping packs as the final step in your evening routine, after all other products have been absorbed. Use a thin, even layer and allow it to absorb completely before going to bed. Some sleeping packs are designed to be washed off in the morning, while others can be left on and followed by your regular morning routine.

The frequency of sleeping pack use depends on your skin's needs and tolerance. Start with 1 to 2 times per week and adjust based on how your skin responds. Those with oily or acne-prone skin should choose lightweight, non-comedogenic formulations to avoid clogging pores.

Routine Customization Guide

This multi-step routine provides flexibility and benefits, and not every step needs to be used daily or by every individual. Understanding how to customize this routine based on your specific needs, skin type, and lifestyle is crucial for achieving optimal results without overwhelming your skin or your schedule.

Daily Core Routine

The daily core routine consists of the essential steps that should be performed every day: oil cleanser (evening), water-based cleanser, toner, treatments/serums, moisturizer, and sunscreen (morning). These six steps provide the foundation of effective skincare and address the basic needs of cleansing, hydrating, treating, and protecting the skin.

Weekly Enhancement Steps

Exfoliation, sheet masks and cleansing masks should be used 1-3 times per week based on your skin's needs and tolerance. These steps provide intensive treatment and can be adjusted seasonally or based on specific skin concerns that arise.

Boosting Steps

Eye cream, moisturizing mist, facial oils, gua-sha and sleeping packs are optional steps that can provide additional benefits but are not essential for everyone. These steps can be added based on specific concerns or preferences.

Skin Type Customization

For oily skin, focus on lightweight, gel-based formulations and include BHA exfoliation and clay-based cleansing masks. Skip or use minimal facial oil, and choose non-comedogenic products throughout the routine.

For dry skin, emphasize hydrating steps like the 7-skin method with toner, facial mists, and sleeping packs. Include facial oils and choose cream-based moisturizers with ceramides and fatty acids.

For sensitive skin, introduce new steps gradually and choose fragrance-free, hypoallergenic formulations. Focus on gentle, soothing ingredients and avoid high concentrations of active ingredients.

For combination skin, consider using different products on different areas of the face, or alternating between formulations designed for oily and dry skin based on seasonal changes.

Timing and Application Techniques

The timing of your skincare routine can significantly impact its effectiveness. Morning routines should focus on protection and preparation for the day ahead, while evening routines can include more intensive treatments and repair-focused ingredients.

Allow adequate time between steps for absorption—rushing the process can reduce effectiveness and increase the risk of pilling. Generally, wait 30-60 seconds between water-based products and 2-3 minutes before applying oil-based products or sunscreen.

The patting technique helps maximize absorption while providing gentle stimulation that can improve circulation. Use your palms or fingertips to gently pat products into the skin rather than rubbing or pulling, which can cause irritation or premature aging.

Seasonal Adjustments

Your enhanced skincare routine should evolve with the seasons and environmental conditions to address changing skin needs effectively. Environmental factors such as humidity, temperature, air quality, and UV intensity all impact skin health and should influence your product choices and routine frequency.

Winter Adaptations

Winter typically requires richer, more occlusive products to combat dry air and indoor heating. Increase the frequency of hydrating steps like facial mists and sleeping packs, and consider switching to cream-based moisturizers even if you typically use lighter formulations. The low humidity of winter air can cause increased transepidermal water loss, making hydrating essences and facial oils particularly beneficial.

Cleansing masks should be used less frequently in winter, as the skin's barrier function may be compromised by harsh weather conditions. Focus on hydrating and nourishing masks rather than deep-cleansing clay masks. Exfoliation frequency may also need to be reduced to prevent over-sensitizing already stressed skin.

Summer Modifications

Summer's increased humidity and heat may call for lighter, more hydrating formulations that won't feel heavy or contribute to excess oil production. Gel-based moisturizers, lightweight essences, and refreshing facial mists become particularly valuable during hot weather.

Increase the frequency of cleansing masks to address increased oil production and environmental pollutants that can accumulate on the skin during summer activities. BHA exfoliation may be more beneficial than AHA exfoliation during summer, as BHAs are oil-soluble and can better address increased sebum production.

Sunscreen becomes even more critical during summer, and you may need to switch to higher SPF formulations or more water-resistant options if you'll be spending extended time outdoors or participating in water activities.

Spring and Fall Transitions

Transitional seasons can trigger sensitivity as the skin adjusts to changing conditions. During these times, focus on gentle, barrier-supporting products and avoid introducing new active ingredients that might cause irritation. This is an ideal time to gradually introduce new products or adjust the frequency of treatment steps.

Spring is often considered the best time to introduce new active ingredients like retinol or higher concentrations of acids, as the skin will have time to build tolerance before the more challenging summer sun exposure. Fall is an excellent time to focus on repair and renewal after summer sun exposure, making it ideal for introducing brightening treatments and more intensive anti-aging products.

Environmental Adaptations

Urban environments with high pollution levels may require additional antioxidant protection and more frequent deep cleansing. Consider adding antioxidant-rich serums, increasing the frequency of cleansing masks, and ensuring thorough double cleansing to remove pollutant particles that can accumulate on the skin.

Air travel and air-conditioned environments can be particularly dehydrating, making facial mists and hydrating essences especially valuable. Consider carrying a travel-size facial mist for use during flights or in dry office environments.

Building Your Personalized Routine

The key to successful enhanced skincare is thoughtful customization based on your individual skin needs, lifestyle, preferences, and goals. The multi-step routine provides a comprehensive framework, but the art lies in selecting and combining the steps that will provide the greatest benefit for your unique situation.

Assessment and Goal Setting

Begin by honestly assessing your current skin condition, primary concerns, and lifestyle constraints. Are you dealing with acne, aging, hyperpigmentation, sensitivity, or dehydration? How much time can you realistically dedicate to skincare every morning and night? What is your budget for products, and how important is the sensorial experience of your routine?

Set realistic, specific goals for your skincare routine. Rather than aiming for "perfect skin", focus on achievable objectives like "reduce the appearance of fine lines around my eyes" or "achieve more even skin tone". This approach helps you select the most appropriate steps and products while maintaining realistic expectations.

Gradual Implementation Strategy

Avoid the temptation to implement all desired changes to your routine immediately. Start with your current routine or the core routine (cleanser, toner, treatment, moisturizer, sunscreen) and introduce new steps or ingredients after your skin has adjusted, or wait 1-2 weeks. Keep in mind that most changes will take at least 6 weeks to see the effect. Also, avoid introducing many new active ingredients at the same time. This gradual approach allows you to assess how your skin responds to each addition and identify which steps or active ingredients provide the most noticeable benefits.

Keep a simple skincare journal noting which products and steps you use each day and any changes in your skin's appearance or feel. This record will help you identify patterns and optimize your routine over time.

Product Selection Principles

When selecting products for your enhanced routine, prioritize quality over quantity. It's better to have fewer, high-quality products that work well together than many mediocre products that may conflict or provide redundant benefits. Research ingredients and choose products with proven efficacy and appropriate concentrations for your skin type and concerns.

Consider the overall balance of your routine. If you're using multiple active ingredients, ensure they're compatible and that you're not overwhelming your skin. Balance active treatments with soothing, hydrating steps to maintain skin barrier health.

Routine Flexibility and Adaptation

Build flexibility into your routine to accommodate varying schedules, skin needs, and life circumstances. Develop a "quick routine" for busy days that includes only the most essential steps, and a "full routine" for when you have more time and want to enjoy the complete experience.

Be prepared to adjust your routine based on hormonal changes, stress levels, travel, illness, or other factors that can affect your skin. The enhanced routine's modularity makes it easy to add or remove steps as needed without disrupting the overall effectiveness.

Long-term Maintenance and Evolution

Remember that skincare is a long-term commitment, and your routine should evolve as your skin changes with age, seasons, and life circumstances. What works at 25 may not work at 35, and what works in winter may not work in summer. Embrace this evolution as part of the journey toward optimal skin health.

Regularly reassess your routine's effectiveness and be willing to make changes when products are no longer serving your needs. Stay informed about new ingredients and formulations, but avoid the temptation to constantly chase the latest trends at the expense of consistency with proven products.

The Mindfulness Aspect

The enhanced skincare routine offers an opportunity for daily mindfulness and self-care that extends beyond the physical benefits to the skin. Use this time to connect with yourself, practice gratitude, and create a sense of ritual and routine that supports your overall well-being.

The act of caring for your skin can become a form of meditation, helping you start and end each day with intention and self-compassion. This mindful approach to skincare often leads to better consistency and greater satisfaction with the routine, regardless of the specific products used.

CHAPTER 9:
POWER INGREDIENTS:
Traditional Wisdom and Modern Innovations

Traditional Wisdom Meets Modern Science

Asian skincare's greatest strength lies in its ability to bridge ancient wisdom with cutting-edge scientific research, creating formulations that honor traditional knowledge while delivering proven results. The power ingredients that have defined Asian beauty for centuries—ginseng, green tea, and rice water—continue to play central roles in modern formulations, validated by extensive research that confirms their remarkable benefits for skin health and appearance.

These traditional and modern ingredients represent more than just marketing appeal; they embody thousands of years of empirical knowledge about what works for skin health. Asian culture has long recognized the connection between internal wellness and external beauty, leading to the use of ingredients that provide both nutritional and topical benefits. Modern scientific analysis has revealed the complex biochemical mechanisms behind these traditional remedies, explaining why they have remained popular across generations [39].

The Asian approach to incorporating traditional ingredients into modern skincare involves sophisticated extraction techniques, standardization of active compounds, and innovative delivery systems that maximize bioavailability while maintaining the gentle, holistic benefits that made these ingredients valuable in the first place. This marriage of tradition and innovation has created some of the most effective and beloved skincare ingredients in the world.

Ginseng: The Root of Vitality

Ginseng has been revered for over 2,000 years as a powerful adaptogen and healing herb. In Asian culture, ginseng is considered the "king of herbs," prized for its ability to restore vitality, enhance longevity, and promote overall wellness. The translation of these internal benefits to topical skincare has made ginseng one of the most researched and effective anti-aging ingredients in the Asian beauty industry.

The Science Behind Ginseng's Anti-Aging Properties

Ginseng's remarkable anti-aging effects stem from its rich concentration of ginsenosides, unique saponin compounds that provide potent antioxidant, anti-inflammatory, and collagen-stimulating properties. Research has identified over 40 different ginsenosides in red ginseng, each contributing to the ingredient's comprehensive anti-aging benefits.

Ginsenoside Rb1, one of the most abundant and well-studied compounds, has been shown to stimulate collagen synthesis by activating fibroblasts, the cells responsible for producing the structural proteins that keep skin firm and elastic. Clinical studies have demonstrated that topical application of ginsenoside Rb1 can increase collagen production by up to 60% over a 12-week period [40].

Ginsenoside Rg1 provides powerful antioxidant protection, neutralizing free radicals that contribute to premature aging and cellular damage. This compound has been shown to be more effective than vitamin E in protecting skin cells from oxidative stress, making it particularly valuable for preventing environmental aging.

Ginseng's Circulation-Boosting Benefits

One of ginseng's most valuable properties for skincare is its ability to improve microcirculation, bringing nutrients to skin cells while helping remove waste products. This enhanced circulation contributes to the healthy glow that ginseng-containing products are famous for producing.

Improved circulation also supports the skin's natural repair and regeneration processes, helping to accelerate healing and renewal. This makes ginseng particularly beneficial for mature skin, stressed skin, and those recovering from environmental damage or skin treatments.

The circulation-boosting effects of ginseng can be enhanced through massage application techniques that stimulate blood flow while delivering the active compounds. Asian skincare routines often emphasize gentle massage when applying ginseng-containing products to maximize these circulation benefits.

Clinical Evidence and Research

Extensive clinical research has validated ginseng's effectiveness for anti-aging skincare. A landmark study published in the Journal of Ginseng Research found that participants using ginseng-containing skincare products showed significant improvements in skin elasticity, hydration, and overall appearance after 12 weeks of use [41].

Another study focusing specifically on red ginseng extract demonstrated that topical application could reduce the appearance of fine lines by an average of 27% and improve skin firmness by 23% over an 8-week period. These results were attributed to ginseng's ability to stimulate collagen production and improve skin barrier function [42].

Research has also shown that ginseng can help protect against UV-induced damage and may even help repair existing photodamage. This photoprotective effect, combined with its anti-aging properties, makes ginseng an excellent ingredient for comprehensive anti-aging skincare routines.

Green Tea: The Antioxidant Powerhouse

Green tea's claim to fame lies in its exceptional concentration of epigallocatechin gallate (EGCG), which provides antioxidant protection 25-100 times more potent than vitamins C and E. This makes green tea the ultimate environmental shield in skincare, offering unparalleled protection against pollution, UV damage, and free radical assault [43].

The Polyphenol Profile of Green Tea

Green tea contains four main catechins: epicatechin (EC), epicatechin gallate (ECG), epigallocatechin (EGC), and epigallocatechin gallate (EGCG). EGCG is the most abundant and potent of these compounds, comprising 50-80% of the total catechin content in high-quality green tea extracts.

EGCG's antioxidant capacity is approximately 25-100 times more potent than vitamins C and E, making it one of the most powerful antioxidants available for topical skincare use. This exceptional antioxidant activity helps protect skin cells from free radical damage caused by UV exposure, pollution, and other environmental stressors [44].

The synergistic effects of multiple catechins working together provide more comprehensive protection than any single compound alone. This is why whole green tea extracts are often more effective than isolated EGCG, demonstrating the wisdom of traditional whole-plant approaches to skincare.

Photoprotective Benefits and Pore Refinement

While green tea cannot replace sunscreen, its unique ability to absorb UV radiation and neutralize sun-generated free radicals makes it an exceptional complement to daily sun protection. Studies show that regular use of green tea products can prevent sunspot formation, reduce UV-induced inflammation, and even help repair existing photodamage.

Green tea's sebum-regulating properties specifically target oily and combination skin, with EGCG shown to regulate sebaceous gland activity without over-drying. This makes green tea particularly valuable for pore refinement and oil control in Asian skincare routines.

Rice Water: The Brightening Beauty Secret

Rice water stands as one of Asia's most treasured beauty secrets, with over 2,000 years of documented use from the Qing Dynasty to Japanese geishas' legendary porcelain complexions. What makes rice water truly unique is its fermentation potential, which transforms simple rice nutrients into sophisticated beauty compounds that fresh rice water cannot provide [45].

Fermentation Transformation

Traditional Asian beauty practices recognized that fermented rice water possessed superior benefits compared to fresh rice water, a wisdom now validated by modern science. The fermentation process breaks down complex nutrients into smaller, more bioavailable molecules while creating entirely new beneficial compounds through natural yeasts and bacteria that convert starches and proteins into amino acids, organic acids, and antioxidants.

Fermented rice water contains significantly higher concentrations of amino acids (up to 3x more), organic acids, and antioxidants compared to fresh rice water. The fermentation process creates natural alpha hydroxy acids, including lactic acid and glycolic acid, that provide gentle exfoliation and brightening benefits without the irritation potential of synthetic acids [46].

The Pitera Revolution

Pitera, the legendary ingredient that built SK-II's reputation, represents the pinnacle of fermented rice technology. Derived from a specific strain of yeast (Galactomyces ferment filtrate) used in sake production, Pitera contains over 50 beneficial compounds including amino acids, minerals, vitamins, and organic acids. The discovery came from observing sake brewers' remarkably soft, youthful hands—a testament to the transformative power of fermented rice compounds.

Nutritional Profile and Brightening Mechanisms

Rice water's effectiveness stems from its rich composition containing B vitamins (particularly inositol and biotin), vitamin E, minerals (potassium, magnesium, zinc), amino acids, and antioxidants. Ferulic acid provides protection against environmental damage while helping prevent hyperpigmentation, working synergistically with other rice-derived antioxidants.

Rice water's brightening effects operate through multiple complementary pathways. Natural kojic acid provides gentle tyrosinase inhibition, helping to prevent and fade dark spots without irritation. Arbutin, naturally present in fermented rice products, provides additional tyrosinase inhibition through a different mechanism, creating synergistic brightening effects. The gentle enzymatic exfoliation helps accelerate the natural shedding of pigmented skin cells while promoting healthy cell turnover [47].

pH Harmony and Modern Applications

One of rice water's most valuable characteristics is its natural pH compatibility with healthy skin (5.5-6.5), closely matching the skin's acid mantle and making it exceptionally gentle while delivering brightening benefits. This pH compatibility allows for effective delivery of active compounds without compromising skin health, explaining its historical use for achieving luminous complexions.

Contemporary skincare has refined traditional rice water through advanced fermentation techniques and innovative delivery systems. Modern formulations often combine multiple fermentation strains while time-release systems allow sustained delivery of active compounds throughout the day, maximizing brightening and hydrating benefits.

Aloe Vera: The Plant of Immortality

Aloe vera's distinctive advantage lies in its immediate cooling and pain-relieving properties, combined with acemannan—a unique polysaccharide that provides immune-stimulating and wound-healing benefits found in no other plant. This combination makes aloe vera the ultimate first-aid ingredient for irritated, inflamed, or sun-damaged skin [48].

Acemannan's Unique Power

Acemannan, aloe vera's signature compound, stimulates macrophage activity and enhances wound healing through mechanisms that other plant polysaccharides cannot replicate. This compound is responsible for aloe vera's ability to reduce burn healing time by up to 9 days compared to conventional treatments [49].

The gel's 99% water content, combined with its 1% concentrated bioactives, creates a unique delivery system that provides immediate cooling relief while delivering therapeutic compounds to deeper skin layers. This dual-action mechanism explains aloe vera's effectiveness for both immediate symptom relief and long-term healing.

Instant Relief Specialist

Aloe vera's immediate cooling effect, combined with its anti-inflammatory enzymes like bradykinase, provides rapid relief from pain and inflammation. This makes it particularly valuable for treating sunburn, minor injuries, and acute skin irritation where immediate comfort is needed alongside healing support.

Tea Tree Oil: The Terpinen-4-ol Specialist

Tea tree oil's therapeutic power comes specifically from its 30-48% concentration of terpinen-4-ol, a compound that provides targeted antimicrobial and anti-inflammatory effects particularly effective against Cutibacterium acnes—the primary bacteria responsible for acne development [50].

Terpinen-4-ol Precision

Unlike broad-spectrum antimicrobials, terpinen-4-ol specifically targets acne-causing bacteria while being gentle enough for regular use. Clinical studies show that 5% tea tree oil gel equals the effectiveness of 5% benzoyl peroxide for acne treatment, but with significantly fewer side effects including less dryness, irritation, and burning [51].

The oil's ability to penetrate deeply into pores while providing antimicrobial protection makes it particularly effective for preventing the bacterial overgrowth that leads to inflammatory acne. This deep-penetrating action, combined with sebum regulation, addresses multiple acne-causing factors simultaneously.

Acne-Specific Benefits

Tea tree oil's effectiveness against antibiotic-resistant bacteria, including MRSA, makes it particularly valuable in an era of increasing bacterial resistance. The oil's ability to disrupt microbial cell membranes while reducing inflammatory mediator production creates optimal conditions for acne healing without the harsh effects of synthetic treatments [52].

Calendula: The Gentle Healer

Calendula officinalis, commonly known as pot marigold, stands apart in the skincare world for its exceptional gentleness combined with effective healing properties. This bright orange flower has been treasured for over 1,000 years, but what makes calendula truly unique is its unparalleled safety profile—making it suitable for even the most sensitive skin, including babies and those with reactive skin conditions [53].

The Gentle Power of Triterpenes

Calendula's therapeutic effects come primarily from its triterpenes, particularly faradiol and its esters, which provide anti-inflammatory and wound-healing benefits without the irritation potential of stronger actives. Unlike many botanical ingredients, calendula's active compounds work gently, making it ideal for long-term use and sensitive skin applications [54].

The flower also contains unique flavonoids like quercetin and rutin, along with carotenoids that give calendula its distinctive color. These compounds provide antioxidant protection while supporting the skin's natural healing processes through gentle, non-irritating mechanisms.

Exceptional Safety

What truly sets calendula apart is its remarkable safety record. Clinical studies consistently show that calendula extracts are well-tolerated even by individuals with conditions like eczema or dermatitis, where most other ingredients would cause irritation. This exceptional gentleness has made calendula a cornerstone of sensitive and pediatric skincare, with extensive research validating its safety and effectiveness for treating diaper rash, minor cuts, and other common skin problems.

Research demonstrates that calendula is non-comedogenic, non-sensitizing, and rarely causes allergic reactions, making it an excellent choice for those with multiple sensitivities or reactive skin who need effective treatment without risk of adverse reactions. This safety profile extends to its use during pregnancy and breastfeeding, where many other active ingredients are contraindicated.

Snail Mucin: The Regenerative Marvel

Snail mucin represents K-beauty's most innovative ingredient discovery, transforming an unusual natural secretion into a sophisticated regenerative powerhouse. What makes snail mucin truly unique is its complex biological composition that mirrors many of the compounds naturally found in healthy human skin, creating exceptional biocompatibility and effectiveness [55].

Unique Regenerative Composition

Unlike other hydrating ingredients, snail mucin contains a sophisticated mixture of growth factors, glycoproteins, and natural hyaluronic acid that work synergistically to stimulate genuine skin regeneration. The presence of allantoin provides gentle exfoliation while promoting cell renewal, creating a unique combination of immediate hydration and long-term skin improvement.

The glycoproteins in snail mucin are particularly noteworthy, as they create a protective film on the skin surface while delivering bioactive compounds to deeper layers. This dual-action mechanism provides both immediate barrier support and sustained regenerative benefits that continue working long after application.

Growth Factors and Cellular Regeneration

What truly distinguishes snail mucin from other ingredients is its natural content of growth factors that stimulate collagen and elastin production. Clinical studies show that snail mucin can increase collagen synthesis by up to 40% in human fibroblasts, while also promoting angiogenesis to support healthy skin function.

Research demonstrates that snail mucin can help fade acne scars, hyperpigmentation, and other forms of skin damage through its ability to promote healthy cell turnover and collagen remodeling. The gentle nature of these regenerative effects makes snail mucin suitable for long-term use without the irritation potential of more aggressive treatments, while providing genuine anti-aging benefits that go beyond simple hydration.

Centella Asiatica: The Healing Herb

Centella asiatica, also known as Gotu Kola, Asiatic Pennywort, or Tiger Grass, distinguishes itself through its unique triterpene compounds that provide targeted therapeutic benefits for problematic and sensitive skin. What makes Centella asiatica special is its specific ability to address acne, scarring, and inflammatory skin conditions through precise biochemical mechanisms.

Specialized Triterpene Compounds

Centella asiatica's therapeutic power lies in its four key triterpene compounds: asiaticoside, madecassoside, asiatic acid, and madecassic acid. These compounds work through specific pathways that make Centella particularly effective for acne-prone skin and scar prevention. Asiaticoside stimulates collagen synthesis while promoting proper collagen organization, resulting in stronger, more flexible tissue repair.

Madecassoside provides targeted anti-inflammatory effects by specifically inhibiting nitric oxide and cytokine production, making it particularly effective for treating inflammatory skin conditions like eczema, dermatitis, and acne. This targeted action allows Centella to calm inflammation without suppressing the skin's natural healing processes.

Acne and Scar Specialization

What sets Centella asiatica apart is its proven effectiveness for acne treatment and scar prevention. The herb's ability to regulate sebum production while controlling bacterial overgrowth makes it particularly valuable for comprehensive acne management. Clinical studies show that Centella can help prevent the formation of comedones while supporting the healing of existing acne lesions [56].

The wound healing properties of Centella asiatica make it especially valuable for treating acne scars and post-inflammatory hyperpigmentation. Its ability to regulate collagen production and reduce excessive inflammation makes it particularly beneficial for those prone to scarring or with a history of poor wound healing, helping to fade existing marks while preventing new scarring for clearer, more even-toned skin over time.

PDRN: The Regenerative Innovation

Polydeoxyribonucleotide (PDRN) represents the cutting edge of skincare biotechnology, derived from salmon DNA through sophisticated purification processes. This advanced ingredient stimulates cellular regeneration at the molecular level through specific receptor activation, making it one of the most scientifically advanced ingredients in modern skincare.

Molecular Regeneration Mechanism

PDRN works by activating adenosine A2A receptors, triggering cellular responses including increased collagen synthesis, enhanced angiogenesis, and accelerated cellular proliferation. This receptor-mediated mechanism ensures targeted regenerative benefits without unwanted side effects, representing a new frontier in evidence-based skincare [57].

Research shows that PDRN can stimulate vascular endothelial growth factor (VEGF) production, promoting new blood vessel formation and improving tissue oxygenation. This angiogenic effect is crucial for maintaining healthy skin function and supporting repair processes at the cellular level.

Clinical Anti-Aging Evidence

Clinical studies demonstrate that PDRN can increase skin elasticity by up to 30% and improve hydration by 25% after 8 weeks of treatment. The ingredient's ability to stimulate collagen and elastin production results in genuine skin rejuvenation, with improvements in texture, tone, and overall youthfulness [58].

PDRN has also shown effectiveness in treating acne scars, stretch marks, and other forms of skin damage through its regenerative properties. Advanced delivery systems using liposomal and nanoparticle technologies have been developed to maximize PDRN's benefits while ensuring stability and bioavailability, representing the future of advanced anti-aging skincare.

Incorporating Power Ingredients into Modern Routines

Morning Applications

Power ingredients can be effectively incorporated into morning routines to provide protection and preparation for the day ahead. Antioxidant-rich ingredients like green tea, and aloe vera are ideal for morning use, providing protection against environmental stressors throughout the day.

Lightweight formulations containing snail mucin or rice water can provide hydrating and protective benefits that create an ideal base for makeup application. The gentle nature of these ingredients makes them suitable for daily morning use without irritation concerns.

Evening Treatments

Evening routines can include more intensive ingredient treatments that work with the skin's natural repair processes during sleep. ingredients like PDRN, ginseng, and Centella asiatica that work with the skin's natural repair processes during sleep. These ingredients can provide anti-aging and healing benefits while supporting overnight skin regeneration.

Fermented rice treatments can be particularly effective when used overnight, allowing the beneficial compounds to work for extended periods without interference from environmental factors or makeup application.

The Future of Power Ingredients in Beauty

The evolution of power ingredients in skincare continues to advance through biotechnology, sustainable sourcing, and innovative delivery systems. Fermentation technology is being used to enhance the bioavailability and effectiveness of traditional ingredients while creating new compounds with enhanced benefits.

Sustainable sourcing and production methods are becoming increasingly important as consumers demand environmentally responsible beauty products. This has led to innovations in cultivation, extraction, and processing that maintain ingredient efficacy while minimizing environmental impact.

Personalized skincare approaches are enabling customized formulations that optimize power ingredients for individual skin needs and concerns. Advanced diagnostic tools and AI-driven formulation systems are making it possible to create truly personalized skincare regimens that maximize the benefits of these remarkable ingredients.

The enduring popularity and continued innovation surrounding these power ingredients reflect their proven effectiveness and gentle nature. These ingredients represent the best of both traditional wisdom and modern science, validated by extensive research and enhanced by innovative formulation techniques. By understanding their benefits and incorporating them appropriately into skincare routines, consumers can experience the time-tested and scientifically proven benefits of nature's most powerful healing and beautifying compounds.

CHAPTER 10:
DIET, LIFESTYLE & INNER WELLNESS

The Holistic Foundation of Asian Beauty

Asian beauty philosophy has always recognized that true radiance comes from within, understanding that external skincare treatments can only achieve their full potential when supported by internal wellness practices. This holistic approach, deeply rooted in traditional medicine and philosophy, views the skin as a reflection of overall health and emphasizes the interconnected nature of diet, lifestyle, stress management, and skin appearance.

The concept of "inner beauty" extends far beyond superficial treatments, encompassing a comprehensive lifestyle approach that includes mindful nutrition, adequate rest, stress management, and emotional well-being. This philosophy recognizes that the skin is the body's largest organ and is intimately connected to all other body systems, making internal health crucial for achieving and maintaining healthy, radiant skin. Traditional Asian culture believes that health is about reaching a balance, creating harmony among your biological systems and your environment. It is absolutely crucial to have a healthy diet, sufficient sleep, good water intake, and low stress as part of your skincare journey, otherwise just treating skin topically will be heavily discounted if your inner health is in disarray.

Modern scientific research has validated many traditional beliefs about the connection between internal wellness and skin health. Studies have demonstrated clear links between diet, stress levels, sleep quality, and various skin conditions, providing scientific backing for the holistic approach that has been central to Asian beauty culture for centuries [59].

The Science of Nutrition and Skin Health

The relationship between diet and skin health is complex and multifaceted, involving nutrient absorption, inflammation pathways, hormonal balance, and gut health. Traditional medicine has long recognized these connections, emphasizing foods that support internal balance and promote healthy skin from within.

Macronutrients and Skin Function

Proteins provide the building blocks for collagen, elastin, and other structural components of healthy skin. High-quality protein sources including fish, eggs, tofu, and legumes that provide essential amino acids without the inflammatory potential of excessive red meat consumption.

Healthy fats, particularly omega-3 fatty acids, play crucial roles in maintaining skin barrier function and reducing inflammation. Traditional cuisine includes numerous sources of beneficial fats including fish, seaweed, and nuts that support skin health while providing other nutritional benefits.

Complex carbohydrates provide steady energy for cellular repair processes while avoiding the blood sugar spikes that can contribute to inflammation and accelerated aging.

Micronutrients Essential for Skin Health

Vitamin C is essential for collagen synthesis and provides antioxidant protection against environmental damage. It's important to include various different vitamin C sources such as fermented vegetables, citrus fruits, and others that support skin health while providing nutritional benefits.

Vitamin E works synergistically with vitamin C to provide antioxidant protection and support skin barrier function. Foods like nuts, seeds, and vegetable oils provide natural sources of vitamin E in forms that are easily absorbed and utilized by the body.

Zinc plays crucial roles in wound healing, immune function, and oil regulation, making it particularly important for acne-prone skin. Include zinc-rich foods like seafood, pumpkin seeds, and legumes in your diet.

Selenium provides antioxidant protection and supports immune function, helping protect the skin from environmental damage and supporting its natural repair processes. Selenium-rich foods like fish, nuts, and grains are important.

The Gut-Skin Axis: Understanding the Connection

Recent scientific research has revealed the profound connection between gut health and skin appearance, validating traditional Asian beliefs about the importance of digestive health for overall beauty. The gut-skin axis represents a complex communication network between the digestive system and the skin that influences inflammation, immune function, and overall skin health [60].

Microbiome Balance and Skin Health

The gut microbiome, consisting of trillions of beneficial bacteria, plays crucial roles in immune function, inflammation regulation, and nutrient absorption that directly impact skin health. Imbalances in gut bacteria have been linked to various skin conditions including acne, eczema, rosacea, and premature aging [61].

Chronic low-grade inflammation, often originating in the gut, can manifest in the skin as acne, premature aging, sensitivity, and various other conditions. Maintaining optimal gut health requires a diverse diet rich in fiber, fermented foods, and various plant compounds that support beneficial bacteria while limiting processed foods, excessive sugar, and other factors that can disrupt microbiome balance.

Stress Management and Skin Health

Stress represents one of the most significant factors affecting skin health, influencing everything from oil production and inflammation to barrier function and healing capacity. When we're stressed, our bodies produce cortisol and other stress hormones that can suppress immune function, increase inflammation, and interfere with the skin's natural repair processes.

The Physiological Impact of Stress on Skin

Chronic stress triggers the release of cortisol and other stress hormones that can significantly impact skin health. Elevated cortisol levels can increase oil production, worsen inflammatory skin conditions, impair barrier function, and accelerate the aging process.

Stress also affects sleep quality, immune function, and digestive health, all of which have direct impacts on skin appearance and health. The interconnected nature of these systems means that effective stress management can provide comprehensive benefits for skin health and overall well-being.

Understanding the physiological impact of stress on skin helps explain why Asian beauty culture emphasizes holistic approaches that address emotional well-being alongside external skincare treatments. This comprehensive approach recognizes that true beauty requires internal balance and emotional health.

Traditional and Modern Stress Management Practices

Meditation, breathing exercises, and mindfulness practices help regulate the nervous system while promoting the relaxation response that supports optimal skin health.

Traditional Asian practices like forest bathing, hot spring visits, and various forms of gentle exercise provide natural stress relief while supporting overall health and vitality. These practices recognize the importance of connecting with nature and maintaining physical activity for optimal well-being.

Contemporary stress management approaches that align with Asian beauty philosophy include regular exercise, adequate sleep, mindfulness practices, and maintaining work-life balance. These strategies help regulate stress hormones while supporting the body's natural repair and regeneration processes.

The skincare ritual itself can serve as a form of stress management, providing a daily opportunity for mindfulness and self-care that helps regulate the nervous system while caring for the skin. This dual benefit demonstrates the wisdom of viewing skincare as both practical care and emotional wellness practice [62].

Sleep and Skin Regeneration

Sleep represents one of the most important factors for skin health, providing the time and conditions necessary for cellular repair, regeneration, and renewal.

The Science of Sleep and Skin Repair

During sleep, the body increases production of growth hormone, which stimulates cellular repair and regeneration throughout the body, including the skin. This nocturnal repair process is essential for maintaining healthy, youthful-looking skin and supporting recovery from daily environmental damage.

Sleep also regulates various hormones that affect skin health, including cortisol, insulin, and sex hormones. Disrupted sleep patterns can lead to hormonal imbalances that manifest as skin problems including acne, premature aging, and increased sensitivity.

The skin's barrier function and hydration levels are also influenced by sleep quality, with poor sleep leading to increased water loss, compromised barrier function, and reduced ability to protect against environmental stressors.

Optimizing Sleep for Skin Health

Quality sleep requires consistent sleep schedules, appropriate sleep environment, and practices that support natural circadian rhythms.

The timing of evening skincare routines can support both skin health and sleep quality by creating relaxing rituals that signal the body to prepare for rest. Asian evening skincare practices often include gentle massage and mindful application techniques that promote relaxation while caring for the skin.

Environmental factors including room temperature, humidity, lighting, and air quality all influence sleep quality and can indirectly affect skin health. Creating optimal sleep environments supports both restorative rest and healthy skin function.

Exercise and Circulation

Regular physical activity provides numerous benefits for skin health through improved circulation, stress reduction, hormonal balance, and enhanced immune function.

Circulation and Nutrient Delivery

Exercise improves blood circulation, bringing nutrients and oxygen to skin cells while helping remove waste products that can contribute to skin problems. This enhanced circulation contributes to the healthy glow that regular exercisers often display.

Improved lymphatic circulation through exercise helps reduce puffiness and supports the body's natural detoxification processes. This can contribute to clearer, healthier-looking skin while supporting overall health and vitality.

The increased blood flow during exercise also supports the delivery of nutrients from healthy foods to skin cells, maximizing the benefits of good nutrition for skin health and appearance.

Hydration and Internal Moisture

Adequate hydration is essential for optimal skin function, supporting everything from barrier function and elasticity to cellular metabolism and waste removal.

Water Quality and Skin Health

The quality of water consumed can impact skin health, with hard water, chlorinated water, and contaminated water potentially contributing to skin problems.

Filtered or purified water may provide benefits for both internal hydration and external skincare routines, particularly in areas with hard water or high chlorine content that can irritate sensitive skin.

The temperature of water consumed may also influence hydration effectiveness, with room temperature or slightly warm water being optimal for absorption and utilization by the body.

Hydrating Foods and Beverages

Asian cuisine includes numerous foods with high water content that contribute to overall hydration while providing additional nutrients. Herbal teas, broths, and other traditional beverages provide hydration along with beneficial compounds that support health and may contribute to skin wellness. These beverages offer alternatives to plain water.

Limiting dehydrating substances including excessive caffeine, alcohol, and high-sodium processed foods helps maintain optimal hydration levels while supporting overall health and skin function.

Creating Your Holistic Beauty Lifestyle

Implementing a holistic approach to beauty requires gradual changes that can be sustained long-term rather than dramatic modifications that may be difficult to maintain.

Building Sustainable Habits

Start with small, manageable changes that can be easily incorporated into existing routines. Adding one serving of fermented food daily, drinking an extra glass of water, or spending five minutes in mindful breathing can provide benefits while being easy to maintain.

Focus on progress rather than perfection, understanding that consistent small improvements provide more benefits than sporadic dramatic changes. Persistence and gradual improvement over quick fixes or extreme measures.

Listen to Your Body

Track your progress and notice how lifestyle changes affect your skin, energy levels, and overall well-being. This awareness helps reinforce positive changes while identifying which modifications provide the most benefits for your individual needs.

Integrating Traditional Wisdom with Modern Life

Adapt traditional practices to fit modern lifestyles and circumstances, maintaining the essential principles while making practical modifications for contemporary living. This might include incorporating fermented foods into busy schedules or finding modern equivalents for traditional stress management practices.

Seek balance in all aspects of life, understanding that extremes in any direction can disrupt the harmony that supports optimal health and beauty. Asian philosophy emphasizes moderation and balance as keys to sustainable well-being.

Remember that true beauty comes from the integration of internal health and external care, requiring attention to both physical and emotional well-being. This holistic approach provides the foundation for lasting beauty that goes beyond superficial treatments.

The Asian approach to beauty recognizes that healthy, radiant skin is the natural result of overall wellness and balance. By addressing diet, lifestyle, stress management, and other internal factors alongside external skincare, it's possible to achieve the kind of lasting beauty that comes from true health and vitality. This comprehensive approach requires patience and consistency but provides benefits that extend far beyond skin appearance to encompass overall well-being and quality of life.

BONUS CHAPTER I:
BARRIER HEALTH & PROBIOTIC SKINCARE

The Microbiome Revolution in Asian Skincare

The discovery of the skin microbiome and its crucial role in skin health has revolutionized our understanding of skincare, leading to the development of probiotic and prebiotic skincare products that work with the skin's natural ecosystem rather than against it. Asian skincare companies have been at the forefront of this microbiome revolution, leveraging their expertise in fermentation technology and gentle formulations to create innovative products that support skin barrier health through microbiome optimization.

The skin microbiome consists of trillions of microorganisms including bacteria, fungi, viruses, and mites that live on and in the skin. This complex ecosystem plays crucial roles in immune function, barrier maintenance, pH regulation, and protection against harmful pathogens. When the microbiome is balanced and healthy, the skin appears clear, resilient, and radiant. When disrupted, various skin problems can occur including acne, eczema, sensitivity, and premature aging [63].

The traditional emphasis on gentle, fermented ingredients has proven to be remarkably aligned with modern microbiome science. Many traditional skincare ingredients, including fermented rice water, ginseng, and various botanical extracts, naturally support healthy microbiome balance while providing other skin benefits.

Understanding the Skin Microbiome

The skin microbiome is incredibly diverse and varies significantly between individuals and even between different areas of the same person's body. Factors including genetics, age, environment, lifestyle, and skincare practices all influence microbiome composition and health.

The Major Players in Skin Microbiome

Staphylococcus epidermidis is one of the most abundant and beneficial bacteria on healthy skin, producing antimicrobial peptides that help protect against harmful pathogens while supporting barrier function. This beneficial bacterium thrives in the slightly acidic environment of healthy skin and helps maintain optimal pH levels.

Cutibacterium acnes (formerly Propionibacterium acnes) is naturally present on all skin but can become problematic when the microbiome is imbalanced. In healthy skin, C. acnes exists in harmony with other microorganisms, but disruption of this balance can lead to inflammatory acne [64].

Malassezia species are yeasts that naturally inhabit the skin and play important roles in lipid metabolism and barrier function. However, overgrowth of certain Malassezia species can contribute to conditions like seborrheic dermatitis and fungal acne [65].

The diversity and balance of these and other microorganisms determine overall skin health and appearance. Probiotic skincare aims to support beneficial microorganisms while maintaining the delicate balance that characterizes healthy skin.

Factors That Disrupt Microbiome Balance

Over-cleansing with harsh detergents can strip away beneficial bacteria along with dirt and oil, disrupting the microbiome balance and leading to various skin problems.

Antibiotic use, both topical and systemic, can significantly disrupt the skin microbiome by killing beneficial bacteria along with harmful ones. While antibiotics are sometimes necessary for treating skin infections, their use should be followed by efforts to restore healthy microbiome balance.

Environmental factors including pollution, extreme weather, and UV exposure can stress the skin microbiome and alter its composition. Asian skincare addresses these challenges through antioxidant-rich formulations and barrier-supporting ingredients that help maintain microbiome resilience.

Stress, poor diet, and lack of sleep can also affect the skin microbiome through various pathways including hormonal changes, immune function alterations, and increased inflammation. This connection between internal health and skin microbiome validates the holistic approach to beauty.

Probiotics in Skincare: Living Beneficial Bacteria

Probiotic skincare products contain live beneficial bacteria that can help restore and maintain healthy microbiome balance. However, formulating effective probiotic skincare presents significant challenges including maintaining bacterial viability, ensuring safety, and delivering benefits without causing irritation.

The Science of Topical Probiotics

Live probiotics in skincare work by colonizing the skin surface and competing with harmful bacteria for resources and space. They can also produce beneficial compounds including antimicrobial peptides, organic acids, and enzymes that support skin health [66].

Research has shown that certain probiotic strains can help reduce inflammation, strengthen barrier function, and improve various skin conditions including acne, eczema, and sensitivity. However, the effectiveness of topical probiotics depends heavily on the specific strains used, their viability, and the formulation matrix.

The challenge of maintaining probiotic viability in skincare products has led to various innovative approaches including encapsulation technologies, freeze-drying techniques, and specialized preservation systems that protect beneficial bacteria while maintaining product safety.

Innovations in Probiotic Skincare

Companies have developed sophisticated approaches to probiotic skincare that address the challenges of bacterial viability while delivering proven benefits. These innovations often combine traditional fermentation expertise with modern biotechnology.

Lactobacillus ferment, derived from beneficial bacteria used in food fermentation, provides probiotic benefits without the stability challenges of live bacteria. This ingredient has been shown to improve skin barrier function, reduce sensitivity, and support healthy microbiome balance.

Bifida ferment lysate, another popular probiotic ingredient, is derived from beneficial bifidobacteria and provides immune-supporting and barrier-strengthening benefits. This ingredient has been extensively studied and shown to improve skin resilience and reduce signs of aging.

Some brands have developed live probiotic products using specialized preservation and delivery systems that maintain bacterial viability while ensuring product safety. These products typically require refrigeration and have shorter shelf lives than traditional skincare products.

Prebiotics: Feeding the Good Bacteria

Prebiotic skincare ingredients provide nutrients that beneficial bacteria need to thrive, supporting healthy microbiome balance without the challenges associated with live probiotic formulations. Asian skincare has embraced prebiotic ingredients as a gentler, more stable approach to microbiome support [67].

Types of Prebiotic Ingredients

Oligosaccharides are complex sugars that serve as food for beneficial bacteria while being indigestible by harmful microorganisms. These ingredients can help selectively support beneficial bacteria while maintaining microbiome balance.

Alpha-glucan oligosaccharide, derived from natural sugars, has been shown to support beneficial bacteria growth while inhibiting harmful microorganisms. This ingredient is particularly effective for sensitive and reactive skin types.

Inulin, derived from chicory root, provides prebiotic benefits while also offering hydrating and soothing properties. This ingredient supports beneficial bacteria while providing immediate skin benefits.

Fructooligosaccharides (FOS) are another class of prebiotic ingredients that support beneficial bacteria growth while providing additional skin benefits including improved hydration and barrier function.

Prebiotic Formulations

Companies have developed sophisticated prebiotic formulations that combine multiple prebiotic ingredients with other skin-beneficial compounds to provide comprehensive microbiome support.

Many essences and serums incorporate prebiotic ingredients alongside fermented extracts and other microbiome-supporting compounds to create synergistic effects that enhance overall skin health.

The gentle nature of prebiotic ingredients makes them suitable for sensitive skin types and daily use, aligning with Asian skincare philosophy of consistent, gentle care that supports long-term skin health.

Postbiotics: The Next Frontier

Postbiotics are the beneficial compounds produced by probiotic bacteria during fermentation, including organic acids, peptides, enzymes, and other bioactive molecules. These ingredients provide many of the benefits of probiotics without the stability and safety challenges associated with live bacteria [68].

The Science of Postbiotic Benefits

Postbiotic compounds can help strengthen the skin barrier, reduce inflammation, and support healthy microbiome balance through various mechanisms. These benefits are often more stable and predictable than those from live probiotics.

Lactic acid, a natural postbiotic compound, provides gentle exfoliation while supporting beneficial bacteria and maintaining optimal skin pH. This dual action makes it particularly valuable for skincare formulations.

Short-chain fatty acids produced by beneficial bacteria provide anti-inflammatory benefits and support barrier function. These compounds can be incorporated into skincare products to provide postbiotic benefits.

Postbiotic Innovations

Fermentation technology has enabled the production of sophisticated postbiotic ingredients that provide multiple skin benefits. These ingredients often combine traditional fermentation wisdom with modern extraction and purification techniques.

Galactomyces ferment filtrate, one of the most popular Asian skincare ingredients, is essentially a postbiotic extract that provides multiple benefits including hydration, brightening, and microbiome support.

Saccharomyces ferment and other yeast-derived postbiotics provide anti-aging benefits while supporting healthy microbiome balance. These ingredients demonstrate the versatility and effectiveness of postbiotic approaches to skincare.

Barrier Function and Microbiome Health

The skin barrier and microbiome are intimately connected, with each supporting the health and function of the other. Understanding this relationship is crucial for developing effective skincare strategies that address both barrier repair and microbiome optimization.

The Barrier-Microbiome Connection

A healthy skin barrier provides the optimal environment for beneficial microorganisms to thrive, while a balanced microbiome helps maintain barrier integrity and function. This symbiotic relationship means that supporting one aspect often benefits the other [69].

Beneficial bacteria produce compounds that help maintain the skin's acidic pH, which is crucial for barrier function and inhibiting harmful microorganisms. They also produce antimicrobial peptides that provide natural protection against pathogens.

The lipids that make up the skin barrier serve as nutrients for certain beneficial bacteria, while these bacteria help regulate lipid production and organization. This metabolic relationship demonstrates the importance of maintaining both barrier health and microbiome balance.

Approaches to Barrier-Microbiome Support

Asian skincare formulations often address both barrier repair and microbiome support simultaneously through carefully selected ingredients that provide dual benefits. This integrated approach reflects the understanding that optimal skin health requires attention to both aspects.

Ceramides, essential components of the skin barrier, also support beneficial bacteria by providing appropriate lipid environments for their growth. Ceramide formulations often include additional microbiome-supporting ingredients for enhanced benefits.

Formulation Challenges and Solutions

Creating effective microbiome-supporting skincare products presents numerous formulation challenges that companies have addressed through innovative approaches and technologies.

Preservation and Stability

Traditional preservatives can be harmful to beneficial bacteria, creating challenges for probiotic and prebiotic formulations. Companies have developed alternative preservation strategies including natural antimicrobials, pH optimization, and packaging innovations.

Encapsulation technologies protect sensitive probiotic and prebiotic ingredients from degradation while ensuring their release at the appropriate time and location on the skin.

Specialized packaging including airless pumps, single-use sachets, and refrigerated storage systems help maintain ingredient stability and effectiveness while ensuring product safety.

pH Optimization

The pH of skincare products significantly affects both ingredient stability and skin microbiome health. Asian formulations typically maintain pH levels between 4.5 and 6.5 to support both beneficial bacteria and optimal skin function.

Buffer systems help maintain stable pH levels throughout the product's shelf life while ensuring compatibility with skin's natural pH requirements.

Compatibility Testing

Ensuring that microbiome-supporting ingredients work well together and don't interfere with each other's effectiveness requires sophisticated compatibility testing and formulation optimization.

Companies often conduct extensive microbiome testing to verify that their formulations actually support beneficial bacteria and don't inadvertently promote harmful microorganisms.

Clinical Evidence and Research

The effectiveness of microbiome-supporting skincare has been validated through numerous clinical studies that demonstrate improvements in skin health, barrier function, and various skin conditions.

Probiotic Skincare Studies

Clinical trials of probiotic skincare products have shown significant improvements in acne, eczema, and sensitive skin conditions. These studies demonstrate that topical probiotics can effectively modulate the skin microbiome and provide therapeutic benefits [70].

Research on specific probiotic strains has identified optimal bacteria for different skin concerns, enabling more targeted and effective product development.

Long-term studies have shown that regular use of probiotic skincare can help maintain healthy microbiome balance and prevent various skin problems.

Prebiotic and Postbiotic Research

Studies of prebiotic skincare ingredients have demonstrated their ability to selectively support beneficial bacteria while improving skin barrier function and reducing inflammation.

Research on postbiotic ingredients has shown that fermentation-derived compounds can provide many of the benefits of live probiotics with greater stability and safety.

Comparative studies have helped identify the most effective approaches to microbiome support, informing the development of next-generation products.

Product Recommendations and Usage Guidelines

For Sensitive and Reactive Skin

Sensitive skin often benefits from gentle prebiotic and postbiotic ingredients that support microbiome balance without the potential irritation of live probiotics. Look for products containing alpha-glucan oligosaccharide, inulin, or fermented extracts.

Start with lower concentrations and gradually increase usage as your skin adapts to microbiome-supporting ingredients. This approach minimizes the risk of irritation while allowing beneficial effects to develop.

For Acne-Prone Skin

Acne-prone skin can benefit from probiotic and prebiotic ingredients that help balance the microbiome and reduce inflammation. Look for products containing Lactobacillus ferment or bifida ferment lysate combined with other acne-fighting ingredients.

Avoid over-cleansing and harsh treatments that can disrupt the microbiome and worsen acne. Focus on gentle, microbiome-supporting products that address acne without causing additional imbalance.

For Aging and Mature Skin

Mature skin often has altered microbiome composition that can contribute to various aging signs. Postbiotic ingredients like galactomyces ferment filtrate can provide anti-aging benefits while supporting healthy microbiome balance.

Combine microbiome-supporting ingredients with other anti-aging actives like peptides and antioxidants for comprehensive age-prevention and correction benefits.

For Compromised Barrier Function

Skin with compromised barrier function often has disrupted microbiome balance that perpetuates barrier problems. Look for products that address both issues simultaneously through ingredients like ceramides combined with prebiotic compounds.

Focus on gentle, barrier-supporting routines that avoid further disruption while providing the nutrients and support needed for both barrier repair and microbiome restoration.

Integration with Existing Routines

Timing and Application

Microbiome-supporting products are typically best applied to clean skin to ensure optimal contact with the skin's surface. They can be layered with other products following the standard thin-to-thick application order.

Some microbiome-supporting ingredients work best when applied at specific times, such as prebiotics in the evening when beneficial bacteria are most active.

Compatibility Considerations

Most microbiome-supporting ingredients are compatible with other skincare actives, but some combinations may be more effective than others. Avoid using harsh acids or antibacterial ingredients immediately before or after probiotic products.

Consider the overall impact of your routine on microbiome health, choosing products that work together to support rather than disrupt beneficial bacteria.

Monitoring Progress

Microbiome-supporting skincare often provides gradual improvements that may not be immediately visible. Track changes in skin sensitivity, breakouts, and overall skin health over several weeks to assess effectiveness.

Some people may experience temporary adjustments as their microbiome rebalances, including minor breakouts or sensitivity that typically resolve within a few weeks.

The Future of Microbiome Skincare

Research into the skin microbiome continues to reveal new insights that will inform the development of more sophisticated and effective microbiome-supporting products.

Personalized Microbiome Skincare

Advances in microbiome testing may soon enable personalized skincare recommendations based on individual microbiome composition and needs.

Custom probiotic formulations tailored to specific microbiome imbalances represent the next frontier in personalized skincare.

Advanced Delivery Systems

New technologies for delivering live probiotics to the skin while maintaining their viability and effectiveness are being developed.

Targeted delivery systems that can deliver specific nutrients to beneficial bacteria while avoiding harmful microorganisms may enhance the effectiveness of prebiotic skincare.

Microbiome-Skin-Gut Axis

Growing understanding of the connections between gut health, skin microbiome, and overall skin health may lead to integrated approaches that address multiple aspects of microbiome wellness.

The approach to microbiome skincare reflects a sophisticated understanding of the skin's natural ecosystem and the importance of working with rather than against the body's natural processes. By supporting healthy microbiome balance through gentle, effective ingredients and formulations, it's possible to achieve healthier, more resilient skin that maintains its beauty and function over time. The key is choosing appropriate products for your skin type and concerns while maintaining consistent, gentle care that supports both barrier health and microbiome balance.

BONUS CHAPTER II: FERMENTED EXTRACTS & GALACTOMYCES:

The Essence Revolution

The Ancient Art of Fermentation Meets Modern Skincare

Fermentation represents one of humanity's oldest biotechnologies, used for thousands of years to preserve food, create beverages, and produce medicines. Asian skincare has revolutionized the beauty industry by applying traditional fermentation wisdom to create some of the most effective and beloved skincare ingredients available today. This marriage of ancient knowledge and modern science has produced ingredients like galactomyces ferment filtrate that have become widely popular [71].

The Asian mastery of fermentation stems from a rich cultural tradition that includes the production of a wide variety of fermented food, all of which rely on controlled fermentation processes to create beneficial compounds. This deep understanding of fermentation biology has enabled skincare companies to develop sophisticated fermentation techniques that enhance the bioavailability, stability, and effectiveness of natural ingredients.

Fermented skincare ingredients offer unique advantages over their non-fermented counterparts, including smaller molecular sizes for better penetration, enhanced stability, reduced allergenicity, and the creation of beneficial compounds that don't exist in the original materials. These advantages have made fermented ingredients central to Asian skincare philosophy and have influenced beauty trends worldwide.

The Science of Fermentation in Skincare

Fermentation is a metabolic process in which microorganisms break down complex compounds into simpler, more bioavailable forms while producing beneficial byproducts. In skincare applications, this process can enhance ingredient effectiveness, create new beneficial compounds, and improve product stability and safety.

Biochemical Processes in Fermentation

During fermentation, beneficial microorganisms including bacteria, yeasts, and fungi consume nutrients from the substrate material and produce various metabolites including organic acids, amino acids, peptides, vitamins, and enzymes. These metabolites often have enhanced biological activity compared to the original compounds.

The fermentation process breaks down large molecules into smaller fragments that can penetrate the skin more easily. For example, fermented plant extracts often contain amino acids and peptides that are more readily absorbed than the original proteins from which they were derived.

Fermentation can also reduce the molecular weight of polysaccharides, creating oligosaccharides and other compounds that provide prebiotic benefits for the skin microbiome while offering improved penetration and hydration properties.

Types of Fermentation Used in Skincare

Lactic acid fermentation, using Lactobacillus bacteria, is commonly used to ferment plant extracts and create ingredients with enhanced hydrating and soothing properties. This type of fermentation produces lactic acid, which provides gentle exfoliation benefits while maintaining skin pH balance.

Alcoholic fermentation, using various yeast strains, is used to create ingredients like galactomyces ferment filtrate and sake filtrate. This process produces beneficial compounds including amino acids, organic acids, and vitamins while creating natural preservative effects.

Acetic acid fermentation, used in the production of vinegar, can be applied to skincare ingredients to create products with antimicrobial and pH-balancing properties. This type of fermentation is particularly useful for creating toners and cleansing products.

Mixed fermentation, using multiple microorganism strains simultaneously, can create complex ingredient profiles with diverse beneficial properties. This approach is often used to create signature fermented extracts that provide multiple skin benefits.

Galactomyces: The Star of Fermented Skincare

Galactomyces ferment filtrate has become one of the most recognizable and effective ingredients in skincare, representing the pinnacle of fermentation technology applied to beauty. This ingredient, derived from fermented yeast, provides multiple skin benefits including hydration, brightening, anti-aging, and microbiome support.

The Discovery and Development of Galactomyces

The skincare benefits of galactomyces were first discovered through observations of sake brewery workers, whose hands remained remarkably smooth and youthful despite their age and the harsh conditions of their work. This observation led to research into the fermentation byproducts of sake production and the eventual isolation of galactomyces ferment filtrate [72].

SK-II pioneered the commercial use of galactomyces in skincare with their famous Facial Treatment Essence, which contains over 90% galactomyces ferment filtrate. This product's success demonstrated the remarkable effectiveness of fermented ingredients and sparked widespread interest in fermentation-based skincare.

The specific strain of galactomyces used in skincare, Galactomyces ferment filtrate, is carefully selected and cultivated to produce optimal concentrations of beneficial compounds. The fermentation process is precisely controlled to ensure consistent quality and maximum efficacy.

The Biochemical Profile of Galactomyces

Galactomyces ferment filtrate contains over 50 beneficial compounds including amino acids, organic acids, vitamins, minerals, and peptides. This complex mixture provides multiple skin benefits through various mechanisms of action.

Amino acids in galactomyces, including glycine, alanine, and proline, provide building blocks for collagen and elastin synthesis while supporting skin barrier function and hydration. These amino acids are in forms that are easily absorbed and utilized by skin cells.

Organic acids including lactic acid, acetic acid, and citric acid provide gentle exfoliation benefits while helping to maintain optimal skin pH. These acids also have antimicrobial properties that can help maintain healthy skin microbiome balance.

Vitamins in galactomyces, particularly B vitamins and vitamin D, support various cellular processes including energy production, DNA repair, and antioxidant defense. These vitamins are often more bioavailable in fermented form than in synthetic supplements.

Mechanisms of Action

Galactomyces provides hydration benefits through multiple mechanisms including humectant properties that attract moisture to the skin and barrier-supporting compounds that help prevent water loss. The amino acids and peptides in galactomyces also support the skin's natural moisturizing factor production.

The brightening effects of galactomyces result from gentle exfoliation that accelerates cell turnover, antioxidant protection that prevents new pigmentation, and specific compounds that may inhibit melanin production. These effects work synergistically to improve skin radiance.

Anti-aging benefits of galactomyces include stimulation of collagen production, antioxidant protection against free radical damage, and support for cellular energy production. The peptides in galactomyces may also provide signal peptide effects that promote skin repair and regeneration.

Other Fermented Yeast Extracts

While galactomyces is the most famous fermented yeast ingredient, Asian skincare utilizes numerous other fermented yeast extracts that provide unique benefits and complement galactomyces in comprehensive skincare formulations.

Saccharomyces Ferment

Saccharomyces ferment, derived from baker's yeast, provides anti-aging and skin-strengthening benefits through its rich content of peptides, amino acids, and vitamins. This ingredient has been shown to improve skin elasticity, reduce fine lines, and enhance overall skin texture.

The fermentation process breaks down yeast proteins into bioactive peptides that can stimulate collagen production and improve skin firmness. These peptides are often more effective than synthetic alternatives due to their natural origin and optimal molecular structure.

Saccharomyces ferment also contains beta-glucans, complex polysaccharides that provide immune-supporting and anti-inflammatory benefits. These compounds can help calm irritated skin while supporting the skin's natural defense mechanisms.

Pitera and Sake Filtrate

Pitera, this complex mixture contains over 50 beneficial compounds derived from a specific yeast strain fermented under carefully controlled conditions.

Sake filtrate, derived from traditional Japanese rice wine fermentation, provides similar benefits to galactomyces while offering unique compounds specific to rice fermentation. This ingredient combines the benefits of fermented yeast with the skin-improving properties of rice-derived compounds.

The amino acid profile of sake filtrate is particularly rich in skin-beneficial compounds including glycine, alanine, and arginine that support collagen production and skin barrier function.

Bifida Ferment Lysate

Bifida ferment lysate, derived from beneficial bacteria rather than yeast, provides probiotic benefits that support skin microbiome health while offering anti-aging and barrier-strengthening properties [73].

This ingredient has been shown to improve skin's resistance to environmental stressors, reduce sensitivity, and enhance the skin's natural repair processes. The probiotic benefits make it particularly valuable for sensitive and reactive skin types.

Bifida ferment lysate also provides prebiotic effects by supporting beneficial bacteria on the skin surface, creating a positive feedback loop that enhances overall skin health and resilience.

Benefits of Fermented Ingredients

Fermented skincare ingredients offer numerous advantages over their non-fermented counterparts, making them particularly valuable for creating effective, gentle skincare products.

Enhanced Bioavailability

The fermentation process breaks down large molecules into smaller, more easily absorbed fragments that can penetrate the skin more effectively. This enhanced bioavailability means that lower concentrations of fermented ingredients can often provide the same benefits as higher concentrations of non-fermented alternatives [74].

The smaller molecular size of fermented compounds also allows for better distribution within the skin layers, providing more comprehensive benefits throughout the epidermis and upper dermis.

Improved Stability

Fermentation can improve the stability of natural ingredients by creating more stable molecular forms and producing natural preservative compounds. This enhanced stability allows for longer shelf life and better performance in finished products.

The organic acids produced during fermentation provide natural preservation effects that can reduce the need for synthetic preservatives while maintaining product safety and stability.

Reduced Allergenicity

The fermentation process can reduce the allergenicity of natural ingredients by breaking down proteins and other compounds that might trigger allergic reactions. This makes fermented ingredients particularly suitable for sensitive skin types.

The modification of protein structures during fermentation can eliminate or reduce allergenic epitopes while preserving or enhancing beneficial properties.

Creation of Novel Compounds

Fermentation produces beneficial compounds that don't exist in the original substrate materials, creating unique ingredients with enhanced or novel properties. These fermentation-specific compounds often provide superior benefits compared to synthetic alternatives [75].

The complex mixture of compounds produced during fermentation can provide synergistic effects that are difficult to replicate with individual synthetic ingredients.

Formulation Considerations

Incorporating fermented ingredients into skincare formulations requires careful consideration of various factors including pH, compatibility, stability, and concentration.

pH Optimization

Fermented ingredients often perform best at specific pH ranges that may differ from optimal pH levels for other skincare ingredients. Formulation chemists must balance these requirements to create products that maximize the benefits of all ingredients.

The natural acidity of many fermented ingredients can help maintain optimal skin pH while providing their specific benefits, making them valuable for creating pH-balanced formulations.

Concentration and Dosage

The optimal concentration of fermented ingredients varies depending on the specific ingredient, intended benefits, and target skin type. Asian formulations often use high concentrations of fermented ingredients, sometimes comprising 90% or more of the total formula.

The complex nature of fermented ingredients means that even relatively low concentrations can provide significant benefits due to the presence of multiple bioactive compounds.

Compatibility and Synergies

Fermented ingredients generally work well with other skincare actives and can often enhance their effectiveness through synergistic interactions. However, some combinations may be more effective than others.

The natural preservative properties of many fermented ingredients can support the stability of other ingredients in the formulation while reducing the need for synthetic preservatives.

Quality Assessment and Selection

Choosing high-quality fermented skincare ingredients requires understanding various quality indicators and assessment criteria.

Ingredient Purity and Concentration

Look for products that clearly indicate the concentration and purity of fermented ingredients. Higher concentrations generally provide more pronounced benefits, though even lower concentrations can be effective due to the potency of fermented compounds.

The position of fermented ingredients in the ingredient list can provide clues about their concentration, with ingredients listed earlier typically present in higher concentrations.

Fermentation Method and Source

Products that provide information about their fermentation methods, strain sources, and quality control processes are generally more reliable and effective. This transparency indicates a commitment to quality and scientific rigor.

Traditional fermentation methods often produce more complex and beneficial ingredient profiles compared to rapid industrial fermentation processes.

Clinical Testing and Validation

Look for products that have undergone clinical testing to validate their effectiveness and safety. This testing provides objective evidence of the product's benefits and helps ensure that marketing claims are supported by scientific evidence.

The Future of Fermented Skincare

The field of fermented skincare continues to evolve with new technologies, ingredients, and applications being developed regularly.

Advanced Fermentation Techniques and Personalization

New fermentation technologies including controlled atmosphere fermentation, multi-stage fermentation, and precision fermentation are enabling the production of more sophisticated and effective ingredients.

Biotechnology advances are allowing for the development of custom fermentation strains optimized for specific skincare applications and benefits.

Future developments may include personalized fermented ingredients tailored to individual skin types, concerns, and microbiome profiles.

Sustainable Production

Fermentation offers inherently sustainable production methods that can reduce environmental impact while producing high-quality skincare ingredients.

The innovation in fermented skincare ingredients represents a perfect fusion of traditional wisdom and modern science, creating some of the most effective and beloved skincare ingredients available today. Galactomyces and other fermented extracts have revolutionized skincare by providing multiple benefits through gentle, natural processes that work in harmony with the skin's natural functions. Understanding these ingredients and their benefits enables informed choices that can significantly enhance skincare effectiveness while maintaining the gentle, holistic approach that defines Asian beauty philosophy. The continued evolution of fermentation technology promises even more sophisticated and effective ingredients in the future, ensuring that this ancient art will continue to drive innovation in modern skincare.

REFERENCES

[1] Khmaladze, I., Leonardi, M., Fabre, S. et al (2020). The Skin Interactome: A Holistic "Genome-Microbiome-Exposome" Approach to Understand and Modulate Skin Health and Aging. Journal of Clinical Medicine, 9(12), 3883.

[2] Elias, P. M. (2005). Stratum corneum defensive functions: an integrated view. Journal of Investigative Dermatology, 125(2), 183-200.

[3] Del Rosso, J. Q., & Levin, J. (2011) The Journal of Clinical and Aesthetic Dermatology, 4(9), 22–42.

[4] Chen, Y., & Lyga, J. (2014). Brain-skin connection: stress, inflammation and skin aging. Inflammation & Allergy Drug Targets, 13(3), 177–190.

[5] Schagen, S. K., Zampeli, V. A., Makrantonaki, E., & Zouboulis, C. C. (2012). Discovering the link between nutrition and skin aging. Dermato-endocrinology, 4(3), 298–307.

[6] Lally, P., van Jaarsveld, C. H. M., Potts, H. W. W., & Wardle, J. (2010). How are habits formed: Modelling habit formation in the real world. European Journal of Social Psychology, 40(6), 998-1009.

[7] Krutmann, J., Bouloc, A., Sore, G., Bernard, B. A., & Passeron, T. (2017) The skin aging exposome. Journal of Dermatological Science, 85(3), 152-161.

[8] Baumann, L. (2006). The Skin Type Solution: A Revolutionary Guide to Your Best Skin Ever.

[9] Pappas, A. (2009). Epidermal surface lipids. Dermato-endocrinology, 1(2), 72–76.

[10] Berardesca, E., Farage, M., & Maibach, H. (2013). Sensitive skin: an overview. International journal of cosmetic science, 35(1), 2-8.

[11] Raghunath, R.S., Venables, Z.C., Millington, G.W. (2015) The menstrual cycle and the skin. Clinical and Experimental Dermatology, 80(6), 481–486.

[12] Byrd, A. L., Belkaid, Y., & Segre, J. A. (2018). The human skin microbiome. Nature Reviews Microbiology, 16(3), 143-155.

[13] Wickett, R. R., & Visscher, M. O. (2006). Structure and function of the epidermal barrier. American Journal of Infection Control, 34(10), S98-S110.

[14] Harding, C. R. (2004). The stratum corneum: structure and function in health and disease. Dermatologic Therapy, 17(s1), 6-15.

[15] Feingold, K. R. (2007). Thematic review series: skin lipids. The role of epidermal lipids in cutaneous permeability barrier homeostasis. Journal of Lipid Research, 48(12), 2531-2546.

[16] Kaplan, D. H. (2010). In vivo function of Langerhans cells and dermal dendritic cells. Trends in Immunology, 31(12), 446-451.

[17] Coleman, S. R., & Grover, R. (2006). The anatomy of the aging face: volume loss and changes in 3-dimensional topography. Aesthetic Surgery Journal, 26(1S), S4-9.

[18] Proksch, E., Brandner, J. M., & Jensen, J. M. (2008). The skin: an indispensable barrier. Experimental Dermatology, 17(12), 1063-1072.

[19] Feingold, K. R., & Elias, P. M. (2014). Role of lipids in the formation and maintenance of the cutaneous permeability barrier. Biochimica et Biophysica Acta (BBA)-Molecular and Cell Biology of Lipids, 1841(3), 280-294.

[20] Schmid-Wendtner, M. H., & Korting, H. C. (2006). The pH of the skin surface and its impact on the barrier function. Skin Pharmacology and Physiology, 19(6), 296-302.

[21] Lambers, H., Piessens, S., Bloem, A., Pronk, H., & Finkel, P. (2006). Natural skin surface pH is on average below 5, which is beneficial for its resident flora. International journal of cosmetic science, 28(5), 359-370.

[22] Schmid-Wendtner, M. H., & Korting, H. C. (2006). The pH of the skin surface and its impact on the barrier function. Skin pharmacology and physiology, 19(6), 296–302.

[23] Cork, M. J., Danby, S. G., & Vasilopoulos, Y. (2009). Epidermal barrier dysfunction in atopic dermatitis. Journal of Investigative Dermatology, 129(8), 1892-1908.

[24] Brooks, S. G., Mahmoud, R. H., & Lin, R. R. (2025). The Skin Acid Mantle: An Update on Skin pH. Journal of Investigative Dermatology, (3), 509-521.

[25] Wang, R., Yan, S., Ma, X., Zhao, J., Han, Y., Zhang, H., & Chen, W. (2023). The pivotal role of Bifida Ferment Lysate on reinforcing the skin barrier function and maintaining homeostasis of skin defenses in vitro. Journal of Cosmetic Dermatology, 22(12), 3427-3435.

[26] Levin, J., & Momin, S. B. (2010). How much do we really know about our favorite cosmeceutical ingredients?. The Journal of clinical and aesthetic dermatology, 3(2), 22–41.

[27] Lodén, M. (2003). Role of topical emollients and moisturizers in the treatment of dry skin barrier disorders. American journal of clinical dermatology, 4(11), 771-788.

[28] Warner, R. R., Myers, M. C., & Taylor, D. A. (1988). Electron probe analysis of human skin: determination of the water concentration profile. Journal of Investigative Dermatology, 90(2), 218-224.

[29] Feingold, K. R. (2007). Thematic review series: skin lipids. The role of epidermal lipids in cutaneous permeability barrier homeostasis. Journal of Lipid Research, 48(12), 2531-2546.

[30] Coderch, L., López, O., de la Maza, A., & Parra, J. L. (2003). Ceramides and skin function. American journal of clinical dermatology, 4(2), 107-129.

[31] Pavicic, T., Gauglitz, G. G., Lersch, P., Schwach-Abdellaoui, K., Malle, B., Korting, H. C., & Farwick, M. (2011). Efficacy of cream-based novel formulations of hyaluronic acid of different molecular weights in anti-

wrinkle treatment. Journal of drugs in dermatology: JDD, 10(9), 990–1000.

[32] Meckfessel, M. H., & Brandt, S. (2014). The structure, function, and importance of ceramides in skin and their use as therapeutic agents in skin-care products. Journal of the American Academy of Dermatology, 71(1), 177-184.

[33] Berkers, T., Visscher, D., Gooris, G. S., & Bouwstra, J. A. (2018). Topically applied ceramides interact with the stratum corneum lipid matrix in compromised ex vivo skin. Pharmaceutical Research, 35(4), 1-13.

[34] Lynde, C. W., Andriessen, A., Barankin, B., Dutil, M., & Humphrey, S. (2014). Moisturizers and ceramide-containing moisturizers may offer benefits for skin barrier restoration and treatment of atopic dermatitis: an expert panel consensus. Journal of Clinical and Aesthetic Dermatology, 7(3), 24.

[35] Choi, M. J., & Maibach, H. I. (2005). Role of ceramides in barrier function of healthy and diseased skin. American Journal of Clinical Dermatology, 6(4), 215-223.

[36] Endly, D. C., & Miller, R. A. (2017). Oily Skin: A review of Treatment Options. The Journal of clinical and aesthetic dermatology, 10(8), 49–55.

[37] Lodén, M. (2012). The clinical benefit of moisturizers. Journal of the European Academy of Dermatology and Venereology, 26(9), 1073-1088.

[38] Prausnitz, M. R., & Langer, R. (2008). Transdermal drug delivery. Nature Biotechnology, 26(11), 1261-1268.

[39] Dattner, A. M. (2003). From medical herbalism to phytotherapy in dermatology: back to the future. Dermatologic therapy, 16(2), 106-113.

[40] Kwok, H. H., Yue, P. Y. K., Mak, N. K., & Wong, R. N. S. (2012). Ginsenoside Rb1 induces type I collagen expression through peroxisome proliferator-activated receptor-delta. Biochemical Pharmacology, 84(4), 532-539.

[41] Kim, J. H., Lee, R., Hwang, S. H., Choi, S. H., Kim, J. H., Cho, I. H., Lee, J. I., & Nah, S. Y. (2024). Ginseng and ginseng byproducts for skincare and skin health. Journal of Ginseng Research, 48(6), 525-534.

[42] Kim, Y. H., Park, H. R., Cha, S. Y., Lee, S. H., Jo, J. W., Go, J. N., Lee, K. H., Lee, S. Y., & Shin, S. S. (2018). Effect of red ginseng NaturalGEL on skin aging. Journal of Ginseng Research, 44(1), 115-122.

[43] Singh, B. N., et al. (2011). Green tea catechins: Biology and therapeutic applications in dermatology. *Journal of Cutaneous and Aesthetic Surgery*, 4(2), 143-149.

[44] Katiyar, S. K., & Elmets, C. A. (2001). Green tea polyphenolic antioxidants and skin photoprotection (Review). International journal of oncology, 18(6), 1307-1313.

[45] Choi, Y. E., et al. (2019). Rice water and fermented rice extracts in cosmetic applications. *Asian Journal of Beauty and Cosmetology*, 17(1), 89-98.

[46] Inamasu, S., et al. (2012). The effect of Pitera on intracellular signaling pathways and proliferation in human keratinocytes. *International Journal of Cosmetic Science*, 34(2), 105-112.

[47] Maeda, K., & Fukuda, M. (1996). Arbutin: mechanism of its depigmenting action in human melanocyte culture. *Journal of Pharmacology and Experimental Therapeutics*, 276(2), 765-769.

[48] Long, V. (2016). Aloe vera in dermatology—The plant of immortality. *JAMA Dermatology*, 152(4), 436-437.

[49] Hekmatpou, D., et al. (2019). The effect of aloe vera clinical trials on prevention and healing of skin wound: A systematic review. *Iranian Journal of Medical Sciences*, 44(1), 1-9.

[50] Lee, C. J., et al. (2013). Correlations of the components of tea tree oil with its antibacterial effects and skin irritation. *Journal of Food and Drug Analysis*, 21(2), 169-176.

[51] Enshaieh, S., et al. (2007). The efficacy of 5% topical tea tree oil gel in mild to moderate acne vulgaris: A randomized, double-blind placebo-controlled study. *Indian Journal of Dermatology, Venereology, and Leprology*, 73(1), 22-25.

[52] Hammer, K. A., et al. (2006). Melaleuca alternifolia (tea tree) oil: A review of antimicrobial and other medicinal properties. *Clinical Microbiology Reviews*, 19(1), 50-62.

[53] Somboonwong, J., et al. (2012). Wound healing activities of different extracts of Centella asiatica in incision and burn wound models: An experimental animal study. *BMC Complementary and Alternative Medicine*, 12, 103.

[54] Titcomb, L. (2025). A literature review on polynucleotide efficacy on skin rejuvenation, and review of the regulatory status and guidelines around polynucleotides. *Journal of Aesthetic Nursing*, 14(1), 9-15.

[55] Bazeer, A. B., et al. (2025). Hidden benefits of snail mucus: A natural skincare marvel. *Biomolecules and Biomedicine*, 25(1), 45-52.

[56] Park, K. S. (2021). Pharmacological effects of Centella asiatica on skin diseases: Evidence and possible mechanisms. *Evidence-Based Complementary and Alternative Medicine*, 2021, 5462633.

[57] Kim, J. E., et al. (2022). Polydeoxyribonucleotide promotes skin regeneration through adenosine A2A receptor activation. *Dermatologic Surgery*, 48(8), 856-862.

[58] Park, S. H., et al. (2023). Clinical efficacy of polydeoxyribonucleotide in facial skin rejuvenation: A randomized controlled trial. *Journal of Cosmetic Dermatology*, 22(4), 1123-1132.

[59] Katta, R., & Desai, S. P. (2014). Diet and dermatology: the role of dietary intervention in skin disease. The Journal of clinical and aesthetic dermatology, 7(7), 46–51.

[60] Mahmud, M. R., Akter, S., Tamanna, S. K., Mazumder, L., Esti, I. Z., Banerjee, S., Akter, S., Hasan, M. R., Acharjee, M., Hossain, M. S., & Pirttilä, A. M. (2022). Impact of gut microbiome on skin health: gut-skin axis observed through the lenses of therapeutics and skin diseases. Gut Microbes, 14(1), 2096995.

[61] Prescott, S. L., Larcombe, D. L., Logan, A. C., West, C., Burks, W., Caraballo, L., ... & van Etten, E. (2017). The skin microbiome: impact of modern environments on skin ecology, barrier integrity, and systemic health. World Allergy Organization Journal, (1), 1-16.

[62] Bouhout, S., Aubert, A., Vial, F., Agullo, P., & Reynaud, R. (2023). Physiological benefits associated with facial skincare: well-being from

emotional perception to neuromodulation. International Journal of Cosmetic Science, 45(2), 123-135.

[63] Grice, E. A., & Segre, J. A. (2011). The skin microbiome. Nature reviews. Microbiology, 9(4), 244–253

[64] Rozas, M., Hart de Ruijter, A., Fabrega, M. J., Zorgani, A., Guell, M., Paetzold, B., & Brillet, F. (2021). From dysbiosis to healthy skin: Major contributions of Cutibacterium acnes to skin homeostasis. Microorganisms, 9(3), 628.

[65] Gaitanis, G., Magiatis, P., Hantschke, M., Bassukas, I. D., & Velegraki, A. (2012). The Malassezia genus in skin and systemic diseases. Clinical microbiology reviews, 25(1), 106-141.

[66] Yu, Y., Dunaway, S., Champer, J., Kim, J., & Alikhan, A. (2020). Changing our microbiome: probiotics in dermatology. The British journal of dermatology, 182(1), 39-46.

[67] Lolou, V., & Panayiotidis, M. I. (2019). Functional role of probiotics and prebiotics on skin health and disease. Fermentation, 5(2), 41.

[68] Duarte, M., Carvalho, M. J., de Carvalho, N. M., Azevedo-Silva, J., Mendes, A., Ribeiro, I. P., Fernandes, J. C., Oliveira, A. L. S., Oliveira, C., Pintado, M., Amaro, A., & Madureira, A. R. (2023). Skincare potential of a sustainable postbiotic extract produced through sugarcane straw fermentation by Saccharomyces cerevisiae. Biofactors, 49(5), 1038-1060.

[69] Mias, C., Mengeaud, V., Bessou-Touya, S., Duplan, H., & Castex-Rizzi, N. (2023). Recent advances in understanding inflammatory acne: Deciphering the relationship between Cutibacterium acnes and Th17

inflammatory pathway. Journal of the European Academy of Dermatology and Venereology, 37(4), 678-689.

[70] Kober, M. M., & Bowe, W. P. (2015). The effect of probiotics on immune regulation, acne, and photoaging. International journal of women's dermatology, 1(2), 85-89.

[71] Pérez-Rivero, C., & López-Gómez, J. P. (2023). Unlocking the potential of fermentation in cosmetics: A review. Fermentation, 9(5), 463.

[72] Yan, X., Tsuji, G., Hashimoto-Hachiya, A., Takemura, M., Tateishi, C., Ito, T., & Furue, M. (2022). Galactomyces ferment filtrate potentiates an anti-inflammaging system in keratinocytes. Journal of Clinical Medicine, 11(21), 6338.

[73] Wang, R., Yan, S., Ma, X., Zhao, J., Han, Y., Zhang, H., & Chen, W. (2023). The pivotal role of Bifida Ferment Lysate on reinforcing the skin barrier function and maintaining homeostasis of skin defenses in vitro. Journal of Cosmetic Dermatology, 22(8), 2247-2258.

[74] Majchrzak, W., Motyl, I., & Śmigielski, K. (2022). Biological and cosmetical importance of fermented raw materials: An overview. Molecules, 27(15), 4845.

[75] Sanlier, N., Gökcen, B. B., & Sezgin, A. C. (2019). Health benefits of fermented foods. Critical Reviews in Food Science and Nutrition, 59(3), 506-527.

www.ingramcontent.com/pod-product-compliance
Lightning Source LLC
LaVergne TN
LVHW051000080826
845145LV00009B/2384

* 9 7 8 1 9 7 1 3 6 6 0 0 5 *